D0720651

THIN
FROM
WITHIN

VEGETARIAN EDITION

THIN FROM WITHIN

VEGETARIAN EDITION

Jack D. Osman

Review and Herald Publishing Association
Washington, D.C.

Editor: Bobbie Jane Van Dolson
Cover Photo: Tom Radcliffe
Book Design: Kaaren Kinzer

Library of Congress Cataloging in Publication Data

Osman, Jack D
   Thin from within

    Bibliography: p.
    1. Reducing—Psychological aspects. 2. Nutrition. 3. Low-calorie
diet. 4. Vegetarianism. 5. Reducing exercises. I. Title.
RM222.2.085   1981   613.2'5   80-24867

ISBN 0-8280-0027-1
Printed in U.S.A.

CONTENTS

To Scott and Brooks,
whose
love of movement
is my
movement of love

ACKNOWLEDGMENTS

The author wishes to express his sincere appreciation to all those who gave him encouragement and feedback during the four years this book has been in preparation: to friends, colleagues, and his best critics—the students—Thank you.

INTRODUCTION TO THE VEGETARIAN EDITION

Some people seldom finish reading books that they begin. I estimate that I finish about one book in ten! I have often wondered how many helpful ideas I have missed out on in the closing chapters.

Just in case you never finish reading *Thin From Within: Values and Vegetarianism,* listed below are the ten key points/concepts/suggestions. The more of these ideas that you can begin to incorporate into your life, the greater will be your success level in the continuous struggle against excess fat.

TEN KEY SUGGESTIONS

1. PLAN! Plan your meals at least 24 hours ahead. Plan your portion/calorie controls. If your situation or condition is such that you must snack, plan nutritious low-calorie foods. Plan for *daily* activity. Plan for some weekly personal growth or enrichment.
2. Eat a moderately large, nutrient-rich, low-fat BREAKFAST *every day.*
3. WALK *daily* to help curb your appetite, burn calories, and enrich and invigorate your life.
4. Cut down and reduce the FATS in your diet. Begin to

learn the visible and invisible sources of these concentrated calories.

5. Drastically reduce your intake of SUGAR. Learn the many hidden sources of this addictive, empty-calorie substance.

6. Drink more FLUIDS that have low calories, no artificial chemicals, no carbonation, no alcohol, and no caffeine. Try watered-down orange juice, or better yet, plain ol' water.

7. S-L-O-W down your eating speed. In doing this, you will be satisfied with less food.

8. Become a more positive, validating, self-approving OPTIMIST. Learn to respect yourself and enjoy who you are now, not what others want you to be. Realize and accept the fact that the battle of the bulge against fat will be a lifetime war.

9. INVEST 30 to 60 minutes a day in reading or reflective writing. Keep a written record in a separate dietary diary or write in your copy of *Thin From Within*. Conscientiously complete all charts and strategies in the book.

10. Solicit SUPPORT from family, friends, and like-minded groups. Open the door of your mind and heart to that Power which transcends the human plane. Ask the Creator of the human body (which is occasionally given to excesses) for power to control it.

WHY A VEGETARIAN WEIGHT-CONTROL BOOK?

Comparatively few vegetarians have problems with excess fat. As a group, they are much more likely to be of normal weight than their meat-eating friends. Research supports the hypothesis that vegetarians also tend to fewer diet-related health problems.

The vegetarian edition of *Thin From Within* was written as a challenge to both the vegetarian and nonvegetarian populations, and to nudge both to a more consistent practice of the principles of holistic health.

Today many persons are looking at vegetarianism as

a viable life-style alternative. In part, this edition was written to assist the interested reader to incorporate the best and latest knowledge available into a vegetarian weight-control program.

The author is unabashedly biased toward the lacto- (milk) ovo- (egg) vegetarian life style. All the fifty-six known nutrients can easily be provided through a prudent use of milk, cheese, yogurt, and eggs in combination with grains, fruits, vegetables, and meat alternatives.

If your diet excludes milk products and/or eggs, please do not be offended by the above-stated bias. Likewise, for the meat-eating reader (fish and fowl included), no one is condemning the form in which you choose to get your nutrients. There is room for all of our diversities. If you are interested in making rational choices, it becomes necessary to know the alternatives from which to choose. This edition presents the lacto-ovovegetarian alternative, and parts of this book will extol the advantages of this life style for sustained weight control and high levels of wellness.

PREFACE

If you want this book to work for you, you must be willing to invest TIME, not just in reading the book, but in yourself. You are worth the hour a day that it will take.

Thin From Within was not written just to be read and forgotten. Unlike hundreds of other diet books, it was written to challenge your present life style and nudge you to consider healthier alternatives.

Research has demonstrated that reading about problems won't change behaviors as effectively as writing about them. *Thin From Within* was designed so that you can write in the book and use it as a dietary diary. Regular reflective writing will increase your level of awareness and grant you insight into those areas of your life-style behaviors that are most ripe for change.

Thin From Within is an *action-centered* book. You must become involved if you want it to work for you. In the final analysis, only *YOU* can do something about yourself. Only YOU can make a difference in your life. Read the book with a pen or a pencil in hand ready to jot notes in the margins or to complete the writing strategies. Add your own thoughts, reactions, and motivational quotes. Make this copy of your book as personal as possible!

In order that you may engage in critical thinking and positive action about weight control, I offer the following pages for your consideration and use. May God bless your journey through *Thin From Within* as you read and write on.

JACK D. OSMAN
Towson, Maryland
October, 1979

THIN FROM WITHIN*

If you are interested in winning at losing, have you considered becoming thin from within? Many of today's dieters are concerned only with what they look like from the outside. They dream of how they will appear when they have reached their goal weight. Little attention, if any, is given to what is going on inside their bodies, much less inside their heads. Becoming thin from within demands that you use your whole being to help you reach your goal weight—your physical, mental, emotional, and spiritual resources. Becoming thin from within relies on your willingness to take a hard look at what's going on in your head and your heart while you are following a weight-control program. The concept underlying *Thin From Within* is that you can get your head together—by clarifying your values—at the same time as you lose weight.

Carl Rogers, therapist and author of many books on counseling, has stated: "All human behavior is exquisitely logical." Surely there are many valid reasons why people eat too much and exercise too little. You can change the external circumstances and even temporarily modify your behavior; however, unless the change is

* If you have not yet read "Introduction to the Vegetarian Edition," please do so.

supported from within your head, even the most effective behavior modification program will not survive the test of time. You need to stop losing the game of weight control and start winning at life.

Becoming thin from within is a *rational* process. Lifelong weight control involves more than just balancing your diet. It requires a lifelong balance of self-direction. Thin from within means you will no longer make excuses for what you are, what you feel, or how you look. Once you have gotten your mind set in the right direction, weight loss that will follow may strike you as the least of your gains.

MOTIVATION: THE KEY TO WINNING AT LOSING

To lose weight permanently, you have got to be motivated. Your degree of motivation is directly correlated to the amount of fat you will lose and keep off. If your reasons are short-term—such as wanting to fit into a swimsuit for your vacation—chances are that you will experience only a short-term water-weight loss. Yo-yo dieting, with your weight fluctuating up and down, is hazardous to your health. You must be willing to commit yourself to a lifelong weight-control program. Don't be alarmed by the term *lifelong*. Almost everyone practices some form of weight control throughout life. To maintain a desired weight instead of going up or down, you will simply be more aware of your program, at least initially. Even as you begin to work toward your desired weight, it is important to set up a nutritionally adequate diet and activity plan that you feel good about and can make a routine part of your life.

Here are some motivational quotes to get you started. Find—or make up—more on your own.

"No" yourself!

What you eat in private
could show up in public

Stick to your diet;
you've got a lot to lose.

The longer your waistline
The shorter your lifeline!

It's when you're on a diet
that the *seconds* really count!

Are you "thick and tired" of it all?

The most attractive curves can result
from three square meals a day!

A minute on the lips;
A few hours in the stomach;
A lifetime on the hips!

It takes a good chooser
To be a good loser

Mirror, mirror, on the wall,
Don't you ever lie at all?

In dieting, the real winners
Are the big losers.
Better waste than waist.

If you eat too many sweets,
You'll take up two seats.

There's only one thin line between
Eat and Fat!

EXAMINE YOUR REASONS FOR WANTING TO LOSE WEIGHT

Rank in order of importance your reasons for wanting to lose weight. Try for at least three distinct reasons. Think your way through to the real reasons, not the fake ones you give other people. State, describe, or explain each one in a short sentence.

1. *I want to lose weight to have a girlish figure again*

2. *To be proud of myself & not ashamed*

3. *So Gordon will be proud of me*

4. _____

Thin From Within

Look at what you have written down. Are these reasons strong enough to modify the eating habits you have followed for years? Will these reasons motivate you to appreciate and meet the need for body movement? Are you willing to walk, even to perspire, regularly? Are you willing to minimize your use of such labor-saving devices as automobiles, elevators, escalators, golf carts? Are you committed to the extent that you will drastically reduce TV viewing?

How serious is your motivation to reach your desired weight? The battle of the bulge is a constant war. At the sure and steady rate of a one-to-two-pound weight loss per week, you must be willing to spend weeks or months reaching your goal. Above all, you must have faith in the program and persist in it. Between 85 and 95 percent of dieters fail to keep their weight off for more than a two-year period. Such a high rate of failure might lead you to think, What's the use? I'll just put the pounds back on again. But you don't have to. It all depends on how carefully you gauge your motivation for wanting to lose weight.

I once worked on a construction project with a man I'll never forget. He held down two jobs. Most days he got only four or five hours sleep, and one day a week he didn't get any sleep at all. When given the opportunity to work overtime, I never knew him to turn it down. An hour before work began he would set up the equipment on the construction site and fill the ice-water containers. One day I asked this father of seven school-age children, "Where do you get the energy to keep going? How do you keep up your motivation?"

"Well," he replied, "some folks *want* extra spending money, and some *need* that extra money. Me? I've *gotta* have it! There are no choices open to me."

If you want to lose weight for some short-term reason, you are probably insufficiently motivated, regardless of how well intentioned and sincere you may be. Even if you *need* to lose weight because of external social pressures or health reasons, your enthusiasm for a lifelong weight-control program may eventually wane. Those who have successfully controlled their weight over long periods of time are people motivated by the internal "gotta" principle. In which category do you belong? Three motivations for weight reduction follow. Circle the one that best describes your reason. Date this chart, explain your motivation, and sign your name.

---

1. I WANT TO *look nice*

2. I NEED TO

3. I "GOTTA"

11-4-81   *Cy.*
    date   signature

When you really *gotta* permanently lose weight, you will definitely have more than "a slim chance in a fat world."[1]

DO YOU REALLY NEED TO LOSE WEIGHT?

"Of course I do! Why would I be reading this book if I didn't need to lose weight?" The popular Carly Simon has a song that goes, "I haven't got time for the pain, room for the pain, or need for the pain." When you realize that most dieters cannot maintain their weight loss over long periods of time, you may decide that the natural mechanism you are fighting is just too overwhelming. Much pain, anxiety, and frustration can be avoided by setting a goal weight that is realistic. If you are a moderately active individual who is between five and fifteen pounds over your ideal weight and you have stabilized at this weight for longer than six months, then perhaps your present weight is your biological ideal. Counteracting this biological mechanism may require enormous quantities of social and psychic energies. Have you the time, the need, or the room for such exquisite pain?

THIS HAS GOT TO GO!

As best you can, draw pictures of yourself at your present weight. Perhaps it would be easiest to start with a stick figure and then add layers of muscle and fat to your appendages. Be sure to provide both a front and a side view.

Looking at your drawings (setting aside your artistic abilities), how do you feel about yourself?

Have you ever really been happy with your figure?

yes
_____

What parts of your body do you like most?

_____

_____

What parts do you like least?

tummy & butt
_____

In the exercise below, list one positive physical characteristic for every negative one.

THIS HAS GOT TO GO   THIS CAN STAY

_____

_____

VALUES, WEIGHT CONTROL, AND YOU

Your values are the stars that guide your life. They light your pathway and give you direction. Taken collectively, your values form patterns that you can steer by, regardless of the situation in which you find yourself. When a decision needs to be made, the person with clearly defined values makes the most appropriate choice consistent with his cherished ideas. Even when faced with many conflicting alternatives, the together person weighs the long- and short-term consequences and then decides on a course of action. Talk is cheap— the valuing person is *action-centered.*

When a dieter has chosen a weight-control program but is making little progress toward his desired weight, perhaps the difficulty is not in the program, but in the *person.* Overweight people who are inconsistent, flighty, irresolute, and apathetic generally suffer from value confusion. They can't see the stars that could be guiding their lives.

"Such persons seem not to have clear purposes, to know what they are for and against, to know where they are going and why. Persons with unclear values lack direction for their lives, lack criteria for choosing what to do with their time, their energy, their very being." [2]

People who are confused about where they are headed will blindly follow almost any plan promising a solution. As the saying goes, "If you don't know where you're going, any road will take you there." Unfortunately, most of the roads available seem to lead dieters around in circles or up and down the scale of yo-yo dieting.

For too long those concerned with weight control have taken only a nutritional or medical viewpoint. The low success rate of these approaches suggests that something must be missing. In the past, doctors and nutritionists have treated just the *problem*—usually with pills and panaceas—and have ignored the *person.* They have rationalized that the diet is the problem—change the diet and you have a solution.

Recently, the in trend for the treatment of overweight has been behavior modification. These principles have been very successful in changing the dieter's behavior. But even behavior modification is not a totally satisfactory approach. Its main concern is with behavior *results,* not behavior *origins.*

The person cannot be separated from the problem. The dieter cannot be separated from the diet.

Thin From Within

Behavior modification techniques affect the diet problem, but not the dieter person. Becoming thin from within involves the *whole* person. It implies that your entire life may need to be reevaluated before you can ever hope to win at losing.

Loneliness, boredom, frustration, fear, resentment, confusion, rejection, disappointment—these are just a few of the underlying reasons why people eat more than they actually need. True, you can semistarve yourself for short periods of time and even reach your goal weight, but unless the root of the problem is dealt with, the weight will eventually return. A "good" weight-control program may help you get thin but leave you frustrated, bored, lonely, and confused. A confused person within a thin body, going in all directions, never knowing which stars to follow, is not the goal of *Thin From Within.* Your task (if you should choose to accept the assignment) is to get yourself together—to win at life—while you concurrently engage in an intelligent weight-control program.

Let's take a moment to record some of the things that may be going through your head at this point. On a separate sheet, write down your major concerns about life, other than your weight problem.

1. Check those that you believe directly affect your weight-control plan.
2. Star the one about which you'll try to do something constructive—*this* month.
3. List at least two things you might do about one of the problems.
   a. _____

   b. _____

4. Write down the name of one person who may be able to help you with this problem.
5. Write a letter to that person and explain what it is you would like help with. (It is often easier to

18

communicate with someone about personal matters in a letter. Once the ice is broken, you will probably gain the confidence to deal with the person face to face.) Be sure to mail the letter.

WHY MOST WEIGHT-CONTROL PROGRAMS FAIL

Since most weight-control programs ask or tell the dieters to give up their favorite foods—for life—the majority of those people who start so eagerly eventually fade away from the fad. The diet program usually dictates what the participant "should" and "should not" eat, what he's "supposed to" avoid, how he "ought to" behave, what he "must" and "must not" do.

I speculate that dieters become confused by all the *shoulds, musts,* and *oughts.* Here they are—intelligent, rational humans—being *told* what to eat! Their choice, and to some extent their freedom, has been taken away. A values conflict results. If they accept the *musts,* they give up their freedom of choice. If they give up their freedom of choice, for how long will their motivation last? Generally, a conflict of values ends in a stalemate of inaction. Perhaps that is why most plans that tell you what to do don't work in the long run and almost never result in permanent weight loss.

The *Thin From Within* plan is based on the premise that you will be more apt to accept a rule or value to guide you through a weight-control program if YOU choose it. The plan avoids the *musts* and *shoulds,* recognizing that there are many workable alternatives. No one says that you "have to" do it his way. You are provided with guidelines that enable you to work out your own program, based on your wants, needs, and values.

VALUES CLARIFICATION

Einstein characterized the age we live in as "a perfection of means and a confusion of goals." Modern life is complex and confusing. The communications media bombard the dieter with suggestions as to what is desirable, what is right, and what is worthy. Today's dieters are finding it increasingly bewildering, even overwhelming, to decide what is worth valuing and what is worth one's time and energy. At the same time, they want the kind of instant results to which our fast-moving world has accustomed us.

People who are unclear about what direction they would like to take in life often lack a system for filtering out the useless and the harmful. Without this filtration mechanism they find it difficult to make choices that are appropriate at any particular point in their lives. A filtration mechanism makes the decision-making process easier by providing a consistent, reliable reference point by which to orient oneself.

It is important that you have a clear idea of what you want for yourself when you decide to become involved in the weight-control process. Consequently, much of *Thin From Within* is predicated on helping you see more clearly the values that guide your life.

The values-clarification process[3] has been charted in the following way:

CHOOSING: 1. Freely.
2. From alternatives.
3. After thoughtful reflection on the consequences of each alternative.

PRIZING: 4. Being happy, proud, pleased; cherishing the choice.
5. Being willing to publicly affirm the choice.

ACTING: 6. Doing something about the choice.
7. Doing it repeatedly, as a pattern of life.

This seven-step process of valuing has been successfully used in weight-control programs. Consistently applied, it has helped people reduce the gap between what they say and what they do—and thus has helped them attain their goal weight.

CHOOSING, PRIZING, ACTING

Once you have freely chosen to embark on a weight-control plan, you can then carefully consider which diet to adopt. In their book *How the Doctors Diet*, Peter and Barbara Wyden elaborate on more than twenty weight-loss plans that physicians themselves practice. Obviously, then, there are many workable alternative plans from which to choose. Which plan will *you* select? What do you *prefer* in a weight-control plan? What do you *know* about the plan that you choose to follow? Before you make your choice, investigate each plan's workability, nutritional adequacy, and safety.

For example, if you consult a bariatrician, a "fat" doctor who treats overweight primarily through prescribing pills (amphetamines, thyroid, diuretics, laxatives, digitalis, or barbiturates), have you considered the possible long-range consequences of this alternative—its cost, as well as the psychological and physiological dependence on drugs that might result?

If a plan forbids you to eat your favorite foods, are you prepared to follow that diet as a lifelong program?

Are you willing to expend the time and effort it takes to decide intelligently on a program that will affect the rest of your life?

Meditate about your answer to each of the following questions:

Are you happy about the idea of beginning a diet?

Are you willing to make the necessary sacrifices?

Do you feel good about the weight-control plan you have chosen?

Have you developed confidence in the plan of your choice?

When you feel good about going on a diet, you are likely to affirm your decision when asked about it. You will, in all likelihood, be willing to make your position known to others.

If you are ashamed of being on a diet, or if you do not affirm your choice when asked, you may have embarked

Thin From Within

on a plan that you do not value too highly.

If you value the need to diet and the diet program of your choice you will *act* upon the plan, not just talk about it. In fact, the plan will direct your eating patterns, and your entire life will be affected by it. If you feel good about your diet plan, you will find it less difficult to practice it as a pattern of life. The most successful weight-control plans do not restructure eating and activity habits precipitately. Over time, new habits are gradually built up that can be adopted for a lifetime.

Intelligently *choosing* a weight-control program, *prizing* it, and because there are good reasons for prizing it, *acting* on it—this is getting *thin from within,* the values-clarification approach to weight control.

---

[1] Richard Stuart and Barbara Davis, *Slim Chance in a Fat World* (Urbana: University of Illinois Press, 1972).

[2] Louis Raths, Merrill Harmin, and Sid Simon, *Values and Teaching* (Columbus: Charles E. Merrill Publishing Co., 1966), p. 12.

[3] *Ibid.,* p. 30.

BEFORE YOU BEGIN

Hollywood and Madison Avenue have saturated our senses with the ideal of the young, slim, beautiful person. This conditioning has so strongly influenced the American mind that many of us automatically reject a partner whose figure is less than optimal.

The male, especially, foolishly believes that only a person with an attractive figure is likely to have an attractive personality. Rarely will he seek a relationship with an overweight woman, even though she is an intellectual heavyweight, a sensuous lover, and capable of the deep emotional intimacy for which he is searching. Unless the male consciousness is suddenly raised, the overweight woman's only chance is to reduce.

Conversely, many a woman is so repelled by a pot-bellied male that she is immune to whatever charms he may possess. In our society, thin is in.

No wonder so many people are obsessed with their weight. Who wants to be rejected on such a superficial basis? The sad truth is that many overweight people come to accept the evaluation made by others and feel that their weight problem cancels out the good qualities of their minds and personalities. They dislike themselves, and see themselves as outsiders in a thin society. Is it necessary to suffer such agony? Can the fat person maintain his sense of security about his self-worth, or does his embarrassment about his physical appearance prevent him from relating to others?

Learning and thinking strategies or exercises are interwoven throughout this book. These have one or more of the following four purposes:

1. To present you with information, opinions, situations, and controversial points of view.

2. To provoke you to think through the relevance of the facts and opinions to *you*, at *this* point in your life.

3. To encourage you to express, *in writing*, your reactions. Since writing provides a relatively permanent record, you may more carefully consider what you really think and feel.

4. To give you the opportunity to reflect back over former reactions, to see if and how they differ from your present responses. Routinely date each strategy after you complete your answer.

ROAMING EYES

Imagine yourself in the situation presented below. Then answer the questions.

You are dieting, but are still more than fifty pounds above goal weight. You've just begun to believe that it is possible for you to be appealing to the opposite sex despite your plumpness.

You're at a party, and have engaged in several conversations. Although they have been neither long nor intellectually stimulating, you're gratified that at least people don't seem to avoid you as they used to. But you notice that in all the conversations people just seem to be going through the motions. They talk trivia and their eyes roam continuously around the room.

Now you are speaking to someone you think is special. Suddenly he/she spots an attractive, slender person coming in the door. Your partner excuses himself/herself ostensibly to get a snack, but actually to make a beeline to meet the attractive person who just came in. You feel you're getting the brushoff.

TO THINK ABOUT AND TO WRITE ABOUT

1. What went through your head as you read this passage? What did you feel?
2. Has this ever happened to you? How did you react?
3. Did you leave the party early? Say more.
4. Alone, back home, what did you do? How did your reaction express itself in your behavior?
5. If this situation were a common occurrence in your life, what consequences might such experiences have on your psyche?
6. List several alternative courses of action that are open to you.

A THIN VALUE STRUCTURE FOR A FAT SOCIETY

Read the following presentation. Then answer the questions.

It seems somewhat inconsistent that society stresses the virtues of thinness and yet saturates our senses with advertisements for high-calorie foods. Most highly lauded edibles are not essential foods; they're more often than not empty-calorie junk foods. If ad men are subtly encouraging us to consume their concentrated goodies, then it would seem that we should be permitted to store those extra calories without being disapproved of by society.

In a society in which nearly 50 percent of the population has a weight problem, who is setting the standards? We can't win! By succumbing to advertising ploys, we submit to excess consumption of calories. When we gain weight, we are made to feel ugly and guilty, because society values thinness. No wonder overweight people tend to be frustrated!

TO THINK ABOUT AND TO WRITE ABOUT

1. Have you confronted the inconsistency described here?
2. What have you done in response to it?
3. Who *is* society, anyway? Have you felt yourself pressured by society? In what way?
4. Have you ever resisted society's pressure? Write about it.

THE CYCLE OF REJECTION

Because society has conditioned us to see thinness as desirable, overweight persons often feel like social outcasts. Clothes are designed for the slender build. Colleges have been known to discriminate against obese students in their admissions policies. Employment discrimination is also common.

Over a period of time, the overweight person's feelings of rejection accumulate and lead to conviction of worthlessness, particularly if nothing is contributing to a sense of self-esteem. When profound enough, these emotions fester into unconscious feelings of self-hatred. Most people's psyches cannot tolerate self-hate, and they protect their psychological well-being by devising defense mechanisms. Some kind of escape hatch is needed to cope with the devastation that is inherent in self-hate.

The trouble is, escape hatches do not solve the problem; instead, they lead to a further sense of rejection as people react to the protective behavior. For example, if the escape mechanism is alcohol, the self-hating fat person may drink to excess whenever he feels depressed about the futility of his life. Food is another popular escape. If the overweight person turns to the kitchen for solace, as he has been conditioned to do, his negative feelings of rejection, worthlessness, and self-hate will be compounded by feelings of guilt because of the failure to stick to his diet.

Alcohol, overeating, drugs, sexual promiscuity,

avoidance of intimacy—whatever the particular escape mechanism, the pattern is the same: people react negatively to the behavior, the person's sense of rejection is reinforced, and so the cycle continues.

CYCLE OF REJECTION*

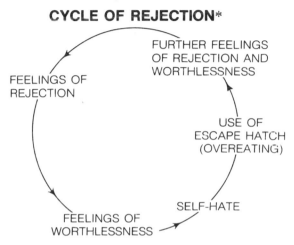

FEELINGS OF
REJECTION

FURTHER FEELINGS
OF REJECTION AND
WORTHLESSNESS

USE OF
ESCAPE HATCH
(OVEREATING)

FEELINGS OF
WORTHLESSNESS

SELF-HATE

OVERCOMING THE CYCLE OF REJECTION

Feelings are real, but they may not be accurate. If you feel hurt because of rejection, that sensation is genuine. It hurts. However, the person by whom you feel spurned probably didn't reject you. The feeling may not be an accurate and objective interpretation of the situation. Before you allow your emotions to overrun your self-image, verbally check it out with the person involved. Don't let the sun set on a low self-image.

When a person feels rejected, it is a totally encompassing feeling. During this period he is bankrupt of any worth, self-esteem, or self-respect. Such emphasis has been placed on the overweight person's most apparent liability—his extra pounds—that he forgets the many assets and equities he has built up in other aspects of his life. Unfortunately, a healthy sense of proportion is hard to maintain in these circumstances. Sometimes the cycle of rejection becomes so intense that it interferes with normal everyday functioning.

Thin From Within

The exercise below is intended to remind you of the positive attributes you may have lost sight of in your concern over your physical characteristics.

On the left-hand side of the space below, list those qualities that you like about yourself. This is no time to be modest or vague. It is a time for a frank assessment of your positive features.

Down the right-hand side print the words *fat, overweight, obese, corpulent, paunchy, plump, heavy,* or any other words that you feel are appropriate to your overweight condition.

THIS I LIKE	THIS I DON'T LIKE

This exercise may strike you as silly, yet to complete it *in writing* is an important step in breaking out of rejection. Look at your list—you have many good and worthwhile qualities. But because of society's obsession with thinness, they're all canceled out, in your mind, by one supposedly overriding characteristic—excess adipose tissue.

As you think, so you are. To break out of the cycle of rejection, focus on your positive attributes. It won't be long before you come to realize that, despite your weight problem (which you have the power to change), you have a capacity for beauty and dignity, the ability to make worthwhile contributions to society, and the right to enjoy yourself and your life.

As your feelings of self-worth increase, you will develop a more favorable vision of yourself—a healthy type of self-love. Many psychologists believe that a true sense of self-love forms the basis of the capacity to love others. Without this cornerstone, all other attempts at love will crumble for lack of a solid foundation.

SELF-LOVE CONTINUUM

If self-love could be plotted on a continuum, where along this line would you currently place yourself? Write your initials at the spot.

   :   :   :   :   :   :   :   :   :

SELF-LOVE   INDIFFERENCE   SELF-HATE

Think about three people you know who are thin or of normal weight, and about three overweight friends. Speculate as to where each of these people might be on the self-love continuum. What similarities or differences do you see between them and you that might be related to your various placements?

Go back and print your name where you would like to be on this continuum, and write the date by which you would like to achieve that end.

List several action-centered behaviors that you expect will be necessary for you to engage in if you are to achieve your goal by the desired date.

1. _____

2. _____

3. _____

4. _____

LIFE ON A NO-RISK POLICY

Simon and Garfunkel had a hit song entitled "I Am a Rock." The song told of a person who built defensive walls around himself for protection against a callous, hurtful world. He renounced friendship, love, and laughter. Hiding out in an idealized world of books and poetry, he managed to cut off all contact with real people. He rationalized his behavior in the closing stanza of the song: "And the rock feels no pain, and an island never cries."

Clearly the individual in the song has built up defenses against intimacy. Perhaps he has been rejected or hurt. As a temporary adjustment, withdrawal may be an understandable reaction to hurtful situations. However, if this attitude of isolation continues, the individual will miss out on many good, reassuring experiences. Perhaps he really would like to reach out again, but is afraid of being rejected. And so he continues to escape, to put up barriers against intimacy.

Have you met withdrawn people with painted-on personalities who acknowledge your presence, yet remain cold, distant, and aloof? The walls they build around themselves trigger a negative reaction in those they meet, which only confirms their belief in the necessity of defenses.

THE RISK-BENEFIT RATIO

Building walls as defenses against intimacy is analogous to the turtle's strategy of pulling his head back inside his hard shell for protection. But even the turtle has to stick his neck out eventually if he ever wants to get anywhere. To reap many of life's benefits, we too must stick our necks out.

We must be willing to take a chance. Initially, it may be only the risk of a smile, a nod, or a friendly gesture to someone. As people react favorably to our nonverbal communication, we may begin to feel comfortable enough to speak up and make a casual observance or share some information.

Positive reinforcement of verbal participation will lead to growing feelings of self-worth and confidence. Eventually we may feel secure enough within ourselves to make other overtures, even assuming leadership roles heretofore unimagined even in our wildest dreams.

THOUGHT CARDS

On a regular basis (daily or weekly) write out a thought card. The writing of regular thought cards is an opportunity for personal growth. (Of course, sharing these personal thoughts with others involves a small risk.) There are three basic rules for writing a thought card:

1. The subject must be something about which you feel strongly. It may be about any topic, of any length, in any style. It may even be a quotation that you particularly enjoy. The thought need not bc restricted to your feelings about food or being overweight.
2. Date each thought you record.
3. Sign your name.

SAMPLE THOUGHT CARDS

"Leaning on a lamppost is not as easy as leaning on a friend."

"It's amazing how things that are not under our control can affect our emotions."

"A friend is someone who knows everything about you and still likes you."

"Don't let old times get in the way of what's happening now."

"Emotions are like rain showers—you can get caught in them when you least expect it."

"He who stands for nothing will fall for anything."

Collect these thoughts until you have accumulated about ten. Then go back over them and see whether they reveal your attitude concerning life in general, or, more specifically, about weight control.

Ask yourself the following questions:

1. Upon rereading, which thoughts would I drastically rewrite?
2. Can I spot a pattern in the ideas that I stand for?
3. Am I genuinely acceptant of most of my thoughts?

4. Have I ever taken action related to the subjects of my most strongly felt thought cards?

If you are ready to take a moderate risk, choose the thought card you are most happy with and share it with a friend.

As feelings of self-worth develop, they slowly establish a stable base for self-love in the finest sense. Feeling more secure, the overweight person experiences a much less drastic need to escape, especially through overeating. As he begins to lose weight, he receives positive feedback from family and friends, enjoying positive reinforcement from a formerly negative society. Warmed by these genuine gestures of acceptance, he is strengthened in his feelings of self-worth. And so the acceptance cycle goes on.

CYCLE OF ACCEPTANCE*

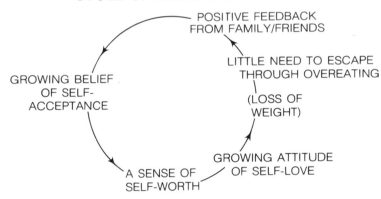

POSITIVE FEEDBACK FROM FAMILY/FRIENDS

LITTLE NEED TO ESCAPE THROUGH OVEREATING

(LOSS OF WEIGHT)

GROWING BELIEF OF SELF-ACCEPTANCE

GROWING ATTITUDE OF SELF-LOVE

A SENSE OF SELF-WORTH

SELF-CONCEPT AND SELF-DIRECTED DIETING

How you feel about yourself will play a great role in how you feel about weight control. The key to winning at losing is getting yourself together—getting thin from within. Once you are sensitive to your own thoughts and feelings, you will learn to do your best to cope with defeats and bad times without slipping back into the cycle of rejection. Your efforts at weight control will be only one part of a well-integrated growth process in your life situation. And because your weight-control program is involving you as a *whole* person, your chances of success—at life and at weight loss—are much greater.

A CAUTION BEFORE YOU BEGIN

At this point in your life, is it safe for you to undertake a diet and activity program?

Be sure to have a physical examination before beginning any weight-control program. Ask your doctor whether you should be aware of any special restrictions in food intake or limitations in activity. People with special problems such as colitis, ileitis, kidney trouble, or heart trouble may be advised not to attempt a weight-loss program.

On the other hand, some persons who think they should be on a restricted-activity program may, in fact, be encouraged by knowledgeable physicians to participate in a mild program of activity. Only your doctor can advise you in this area. His instructions should supersede those of any weight-control plan you may read about.

I, _____, have checked with my doc-

tor, _____, on _____; he has given me his approval to begin a diet and activity program, being cognizant of the following limitations:

_____	_____
date	*signature*

THE PHYSICIAN: IS HE *REALLY* IMPORTANT?

Some authorities feel strongly that the physician must remain the cornerstone of obesity therapy. They insist that the management of obesity is and will remain a medical problem, and that decisions regarding a weight-control program, such as who, when, and how much, should rightfully be made by a physician. The plan, in their thinking, should be carried out under his guidance, or at least with his knowledge.

The other viewpoint is that many health professionals, including physicians, are not qualified in nutrition and obesity management.

And of course, there is the fact that physicians willing to treat the overweight range from the conscientious and highly qualified doctor to the one who simply relies on a diet sheet. And there are even those who deal in lucrative but highly questionable and perhaps dangerous methods.

TO THINK ABOUT AND TO WRITE ABOUT

1. Do you feel that a doctor should be the cornerstone of a weight-control program?
2. Do you feel that many doctors are not adequately trained to handle obesity problems?
3. Would you consult a bariatrician—a doctor who specializes in the treatment of fat patients? Say more.
4. How would you know whether the doctor you consulted about your weight problem was sufficiently qualified?
5. How adequate is your own knowledge about weight control?
6. List at least three sources of reliable weight-control information.

---

* Adapted from M. B. Hodge, *Your Fear of Love* (Garden City, N.Y.: Doubleday & Co., Inc., 1967).

HOW SERIOUS ARE YOU ABOUT LOSING WEIGHT?

Deprivation dieting, the most popular type, can, and often does, backfire. As the dieter approaches his ideal weight, he tends to slacken off and revert to his old eating patterns—often with enthusiasm—because he has had to exist for some time without his favorite foods. When eating patterns are restricted more severely than the human constitution will tolerate, either the dieter will defy the restriction and eat as much as he wants of the forbidden food or his continued frustration will result in neurotic patterns of behavior—sneaking food, deceiving himself, acting irritable.

To lose weight permanently, a person must modify the conditioned habits that caused overweight. This means a sensible, long-term weight-control plan. Nutritional reeducation is what the dieter needs, and this is where most popular diets fail. On a crash calorie-reduction diet, the dieter is generally instructed (somewhat dogmatically) only to deprive himself of certain foods. These taboo viands may fulfill certain social or psychological needs. It is no wonder that these are the very foods craved by the cautious calorie counter once he has won the physiological battle of the bulge. If you are thinking of attempting a very restrictive diet, consider the following.

ON-AGAIN, OFF-AGAIN DIETING

The average American goes on one and a half diets per year, often going on and off with the changing seasons. For some dieters, this approach could mean that health is getting the shaft.

People who lose weight generally gain back much of the shed poundage during the same year. This on-again, off-again system of dieting results not only in frustration but also in possible damage to the heart and other organs. Several authorities suggest that mildly overweight persons should remain that way rather than run the risk of damaging their health by this yo-yo dieting pattern.

An extreme example is cited by Peter Wyden in his book *The Overweight Society:*

"Medical literature routinely notes cases of dieters who have spent years losing and regaining hundreds of pounds in what Dr. Jean Mayer, a noted Harvard physiologist, has called "the rhythm method of girth control." And sometimes the obsession to alternate between extremes of calorie excess and self-deprivation has led to the most tragic results. (The best known example is probably Mario Lanza, the "American Caruso," who once enjoyed twenty-three egg omelets for breakfast. He died of a heart attack at thirty-eight after a lifetime of binge eating and binge dieting during which he dropped, on at least one occasion, 100 of his 270 pounds.)" *

TO THINK ABOUT AND TO WRITE ABOUT

1. How many times have *you* lost weight only to regain much of it?
2. How did you feel about yourself after you gained the weight back, particularly if you had a difficult time reducing?
3. On food-avoidance, calorie-restriction plans, once

dieters reach their ideal weight they have a desire to go back to their old eating patterns and to consume the foods they have deprived themselves of. What are your potential binge foods? What alternatives are open to you in an attempt to avoid this yo-yo effect?

THE "CARBOHOLIC STRAINER" THEORY

Some carbohydrates sugar (sucrose) and refined starches—are said to be the downfall of many a conscientious dieter. The ingestion of the smallest quantity of these carbohydrates seems to trigger a reflex mechanism that signals the eater to go on a binge comparable to that of the alcoholic. This disease has been referred to as carboholism—rendering one's life unmanageable as a result of ingesting excessive quantities of refined carbohydrate foods.

Now picture within each person a strainer, the function of which is to gradually filter carbohydrates through the metabolic process. If the strainer becomes faulty or breaks down, the amount of carbohydrates released into the system becomes overwhelming. Paradoxically, this flooding of the system triggers carboholism—the abnormal reaction to consume even more carbohydrates.

The strainer, once ruptured, will probably never repair itself. Therefore, it is necessary for carboholics to avoid their particular binge foods—one day at a time—for the rest of their lives.

Speculation based on the strainer theory suggests that overexposure to refined carbohydrates, such as those empty calories of junk foods, debilitates the strainer before its time.

Some persons may have inherited a weak strainer and will break down early in life. Others, by continually bombarding the strainer with carbohydrates, eventually will destroy their strainers.

Thin From Within

1. What condition would you say *your* strainer is in?

2. List five foods that have binge potential in your life.

Rank	Food
_____	_____
_____	_____
_____	_____
_____	_____
_____	_____

Circle those that are predominantly carbohydrates or refined sugars.

3. What alternatives could you use to control binge consumption of these foods?

4. Circle the most reasonable of the above alternatives.

5. What course of action do you feel you can establish in order to deal with your binge eating?

DIET AFTER DIET

On the chart below, list the various diet plans or weight-control methods that you have tried.

Indicate the number of pounds you lost on each diet.

Identify each plan according to the following code:

1. Write "Dr." if the plan required medical supervision.

2. Write "$" if the plan cost money for a service or a product (other than a book).

How Serious Are You About Losing Weight?

3. Write "T" for the plan that kept weight off for the longest period of time.
4. Write "Rx" if the plan required that you use drugs.
5. Mark the plan with an "X" if it proved harmful to your health.
6. Draw a smiling face—☺—beside any plan you felt pleased with or happy about at the time you were following it.

Write down the best aspects of each plan.

METHOD	NO. OF LBS. LOST	CODING	BEST FEATURES

Is it possible to extract and use the best features of the plans listed above? Say more.

IF YOU'RE READY

If you are really serious about losing weight, let's make some realistic long-range calculations.

MY PRESENT WEIGHT: _____

MY DESIRED WEIGHT: _____

I NEED TO LOSE: _____

Unless you are grossly overweight—seventy-five pounds or more—it is not recommended that you lose more than two pounds per week. In fact, a pound and a half is probably more realistic. There are several reasons for this. Generally, a weekly drop of more than one and a half pounds reflects water loss, not fat loss. Since the body needs a certain amount of water to operate properly, it will either replace the lost water or operate inefficiently, leaving the dieter tired, weak, and lethargic. Besides, losing more than two pounds per week would require too drastic a reduction in your daily caloric intake and thus place too great a strain on your system and emotions. Finally, when calories are restricted too severely, chances are that your diet will be nutritionally inadequate.

Condition yourself to a long-term program. It has taken you months or possibly years of gradual gaining to reach your present weight. An almost equivalent amount of time will be needed to reverse the process. In estimating how long it will take to reach your desired weight, you must first realistically determine how much you are willing and able to restrict your caloric intake over a long period of time.

To get a rough estimate of the number of calories that you are probably consuming to maintain your present overweight, multiply your present weight by the appropriate constant—16 for females, 17 for males. (Add 1 if you are active. Subtract 1 if you are inactive.)

For contrast, also calculate what your caloric intake

will be when you reach your goal weight.

The number of calories needed to maintain your current weight will change as you lose weight. Recalculate that figure every two months.

In order to lose at the rate of one to two pounds per week you have three choices:

1. Significantly reduce your caloric intake. Eat less.

2. Increase your caloric expenditure through activity. Do more.

3. Mildly restrict your caloric intake and moderately increase your activity level. Eat less and do more.

Authorities recommend a reduction of about 500 to 800 calories per day. *In addition,* they also strongly recommend an increase in activity to help burn up an additional 200 to 400 calories per day. Walking is the recommended activity. Invest 30 minutes or more per day in your walking program.

If after about a month on this plan no results are seen, then perhaps you are one of the 5 percent of the population blessed—or cursed—with a body system that is more efficient and economical than that of most people. You require fewer calories to do the same amount of work as someone who is similar to you in most other respects. If this is the case, then it will be necessary to further restrict your caloric intake (or increase your walking), and reduce the calorie-calculating constant to 14 or 15 if you are a woman, and 15 or 16 if you are a man. After a week or two at the modified level, you will begin to get observable results.

As you begin the program you may be overzealous and decide to restrict your daily caloric intake more severely. Don't yield to that temptation. Too few calories not only decrease the nutritional adequacy of your diet but also lead to hunger pains that may cause you to eat more rapidly than normal. Eating quickly increases the likelihood that you will eat *more* calories before you feel satisfied. Regular meals with moderate caloric restriction will prevent that hunger-pain feeling.

Remember, too, that a more drastic calorie restriction

Thin From Within

does not entitle you to forget about increasing your activity. *Mild activity is extremely important.* Ultimately the choice is yours, but whatever weight-control program you choose, be aware that a combined program of decreased calories and increased activity is the most successful *over long periods of time.* The next few chapters will present information that will enable you to intelligently choose a diet and activity program that will take weight off safely, and keep it off permanently.

PLANNING AHEAD

To lose one pound per week you must cut your calorie intake or increase your activity (preferably a combination of the two) by 500 calories per day. If you wish to lose 2 pounds per week, you need to show a deficit of 1,000 calories per day. Reducing your daily caloric intake by *more* than 1,000 calories per day is too limiting and too drastic a change for a long-term diet. To continue on such a restrictive program for more than 10 days will discourage even the "gotta" motivated dieter.

Use the chart below to predict how long it will take you to reach your goal.

Increase Activity or Cut Your Daily Intake of Calories by	Days It Takes to Lose									
	1 lb.	2 lb.	3 lb.	4 lb.	5 lb.	6 lb.	7 lb.	8 lb.	9 lb.	10 lb.
100	35	70	105	140	175	210	245	280	315	350
200	17.5	35	52.5	70	87.5	105	122.5	140	157.5	175
300	12	24	36	48	60	72	84	96	108	120
400	9	18	27	36	45	54	63	72	81	90
500	7	14	21	28	35	42	49	56	63	70
600	6	12	18	24	30	36	42	48	54	60
700	5	10	15	20	25	30	35	40	45	50
800	4.5	9	13.5	18	22.5	27	31.5	36	40.5	45
900	4	8	12	16	20	24	28	32	36	40
1,000	3.5	7	10.5	14	17.5	21	24.5	28	31.5	35
1,100	3.1	6.2	9.3	12.4	15.5	18.6	21.7	24.8	27.9	31
1,200	3	6	9	12	15	18	21	24	27	30

How Serious Are You About Losing Weight?

The number of calories you are willing to give up each day determines how rapidly your body will give up fat. To lose one pound, you need to lose 3,500 calories. If you cut 100 calories each day from your daily intake, you will lose one pound in 35 days. At this rate you will lose between 9 and 12 pounds in one year. If you cut 1,000 calories each day from your daily intake, you will lose weight at a rate ten times faster, that is, one pound every 3.5 days, or about 100 pounds in one year!

Choose a date when you *gotta* conscientiously begin your weight-control plan. Write it down here: _____

Count ahead the total number of days that it will take to reach your goal weight. Record date here: _____

If you're really committed to this goal, complete the following contract.

Contract

I, _____, do hereby contract to begin a weight-control plan of restricting my caloric intake and increasing my activity by _____ calories daily, beginning on _____. I am fully aware that at this rate, I will reach my goal of desired-weight pounds in approximately _____ days. I further realize that when I reach my desired weight on or before _____, I still must continue on a sensible eating and activity program for the rest of my life if I am to maintain my desired weight.

_____	_____
date	signature

Make a copy of this completed contract and place it in a spot where you will see it regularly—on the refrigerator door, perhaps, or on your mirror.

THE IMPORTANCE OF FRIENDS

Once you feel comfortable with this contract, it is important that you share its contents with a "significant other"—some relative or friend whom you care about, trust, and respect. Ask him to countersign your contract, thereby indicating his support of your undertaking.

If you choose not to share the contract with someone right now, plan to do so in the near future. It is important to publicly affirm your choice to others—to let people know that you wish to make changes in your life. Their support and encouragement are extremely important. If you are shy about bringing up the subject, perhaps your displayed copy of the contract will provoke questions from those who see it.

Support from the people with whom you interact is essential to your success. You need continual encouragement, feedback, and reinforcement. Ask a number of relatives and friends to form a buddy system—a group of people you can turn to by telephone when temptation or depression threatens to overwhelm you.

List at least three people to whom you will send such a letter. When you have written to them, enter here the date each letter was mailed.

Name   *Date*

1. _____   _____

2. _____   _____

3. _____   _____

---

* Peter Wyden, *The Overweight Society* (New York: William Morrow and Co., 1965), p. 5.

GETTING PSYCHED FOR STARTING

None of the numerous hints shared in this chapter will be earth-shattering to you. Practiced collectively, however, these suggestions will easily result in a one-to-two-pound weight loss per week. As you will see, most of the suggestions make "calorie sense." Many of them you can perform right now with only slight modification of your normal eating and activity patterns.

Write your initials next to every hint that you can begin to practice *right now* without any great stress or hassle. Write the date next to the hints you will begin in the future.

SURE-FIRE HINTS TO DECREASE TOTAL CALORIC INTAKE

_____ Accept the fact that weight control is a lifelong struggle. If you let down your guard, fat will creep back.

_____ For the next few weeks totally involve yourself in thinking, reading, and writing about weight control. You must arm yourself with as much knowledge as possible to win the battle of the bulge. Provide yourself with a fairly comprehensive list-

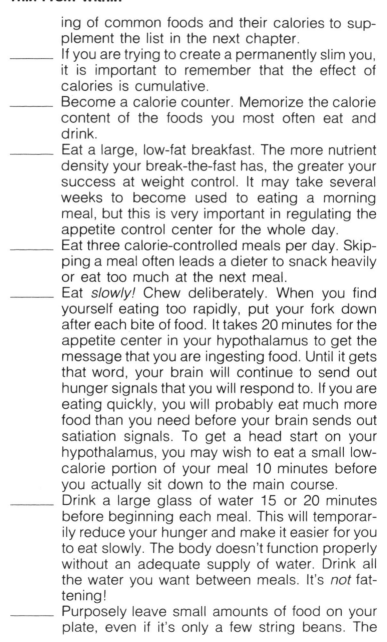

ing of common foods and their calories to supplement the list in the next chapter.

_____ If you are trying to create a permanently slim you, it is important to remember that the effect of calories is cumulative.

_____ Become a calorie counter. Memorize the calorie content of the foods you most often eat and drink.

_____ Eat a large, low-fat breakfast. The more nutrient density your break-the-fast has, the greater your success at weight control. It may take several weeks to become used to eating a morning meal, but this is very important in regulating the appetite control center for the whole day.

_____ Eat three calorie-controlled meals per day. Skipping a meal often leads a dieter to snack heavily or eat too much at the next meal.

_____ Eat _slowly!_ Chew deliberately. When you find yourself eating too rapidly, put your fork down after each bite of food. It takes 20 minutes for the appetite center in your hypothalamus to get the message that you are ingesting food. Until it gets that word, your brain will continue to send out hunger signals that you will respond to. If you are eating quickly, you will probably eat much more food than you need before your brain sends out satiation signals. To get a head start on your hypothalamus, you may wish to eat a small low-calorie portion of your meal 10 minutes before you actually sit down to the main course.

_____ Drink a large glass of water 15 or 20 minutes before beginning each meal. This will temporarily reduce your hunger and make it easier for you to eat slowly. The body doesn't function properly without an adequate supply of water. Drink all the water you want between meals. It's _not_ fattening!

_____ Purposely leave small amounts of food on your plate, even if it's only a few string beans. The clean-plate syndrome has been the downfall of many a well-intentioned dieter. When there is a little bit of food left on the plate, it demonstrates that you have control over your food, not vice versa.

_____ Think and talk about your feelings when you leave food on your plate. The mind plays tricks on us. We begin to think up reasons for eating everything. Talking with emphatic friends about your feelings will often help keep things in proper perspective.

_____ Substitute skim milk (90 calories for 8 ounces) for whole milk (160 calories), or try 1-percent-butterfat-content milk (115 calories) or 2% milk (140 calories). Keep a record of how many calories you saved; then calculate how much weight those saved calories would have caused you to gain in a year. (Remember, 100 excess calories per day will cause a 9-to-12-pound weight gain per year.)

_____ Keep a written record of the calories you save by sheer discipline, as well as those you save by the substitution method. Keep a running total of the calories you save daily. It will bring a smile to your face to know that you are making yourself thinner every time you save calories.

_____ Have someone take your photograph at different stages of your diet. You may want to wear the same outfit each time. Place these pictures somewhere in your book or in your diet diary. This will give you an excellent before-after perspective.

_____ Increase your intake of high-fiber foods, particularly whole-grain breads and cereals, fruits, and vegetables. They will supply additional nutrition and bulk.

_____ Begin your dinner with a salad, but choose a low-calorie dressing and use it sparingly. Regular-calorie dressings may be used, but cut to one-half your normal serving. Below are the calorie contents for one tablespoon of popular salad dressings in regular and low-calorie form. Regular salad dressings are high in fat. Low-calorie dressings are higher in water content. You can s-t-r-e-t-c-h your salad dressing and reduce calories by adding water to it.

Dressing	Regular	Low Calorie
Thousand Island	70	25
Blue Cheese	71	11
French	57	13
Italian	77	11
Mayonnaise	110	19

_____ Reduce your salt intake. Learn to taste food first before you grab for the salt shaker. Reducing salt intake will help you retain less fluids.

_____ Eat smaller portions of high-calorie foods. Form the habit of preparing smaller portions.

_____ Give yourself an advantage by using smaller plates. This will fulfill your psychological need to see a full plate while reducing caloric intake. Try it. It really works!

_____ Cut down on all fats, but particularly those of animal origin. Fat is the most concentrated source of calories—two and a quarter times more concentrated than carbohydrates.

_____ You need not eliminate bread from your diet. Use small or thin slices, thus providing fewer calories per slice.

_____ Whole-grain breads provide significant nutrition, but be careful of what you spread on the slices. Per level tablespoon, jelly contains 50 calories; apple butter, 32 calories; margarine and butter, 100 calories; peanut butter, 90 calories. The latter does contain some important nutrients, however. Heaping tablespoons contain twice the calories.

_____ Whole potatoes are an excellent source of nutrients, but be careful how you prepare them. Minimize your consumption of fat-fried potatoes—hashbrowns, home fries, French fries, potato sticks, and potato chips. Cut down (or out) the butter, margarine, or sour cream on baked potatoes. Cottage cheese is a surprisingly tasty topping.

_____ Increase the amount of vegetables in your diet, particularly the low-calorie ones. Besides providing bulk, color, and essential vitamins, they usually require you to chew deliberately, thereby giving the food time to send its message to your hypothalamus.

_____ Use artificial sweeteners occasionally—if you must use sweeteners at all.

_____ Train yourself to enjoy natural flavors.

_____ If you must drink carbonated beverages, choose diet soda.

_____ Rediscover your taste for that inexpensive, zero-calorie, nonintoxicating drink—water.

_____ Minimize your intake of all fried foods. Whatever you fry absorbs the fat, and at 255 calories per ounce—who needs that grease!

_____ Be creative. Invent and serve nutritious, low-calorie desserts. When it comes to desserts, it's not always feasible to abstain. After all, why should you? Don't eat a full serving—nibble at it, leave some in the dish, or use a smaller one. Desserts can provide an exercise in resisting temptation. Have a successful workout.

_____ Don't eat while watching television. When we are mentally engrossed in something, we tend to eat unconsciously and lose track of our total caloric intake.

_____ Don't fool yourself when you cheat! Calories _do_ count. Be aware of the tastes you snitch during food preparation, and work on overcoming the habit.

Thin From Within

_____ Watch those leftovers! Beware of the "I'll just finish this up" attitude. You may not want the leftover food to go to waste, but if you eat it, it will go to *your* waist. Have someone else clean up after meals. Dispose of scraps by putting them into the garbage can, or wrap up leftovers for immediate refrigeration.

_____ Snacking is not advised, but if you must, save something from one of your regular meals—a piece of fruit, crisp celery, a glass of skim milk. A large stalk of celery, eaten plain, is an excellent snack for the weight watcher (5 calories per stalk).

Most raw vegetables are good nutritionally and low in calories. They also slow you down by making you chew more.

_____ Eat your snacks in the same room where you eat all your meals. This will help you realize that calories in snacks count just as much as calories eaten at meals.

_____ Don't hold lengthy telephone conversations in the kitchen. It's too easy to nibble.

_____ When you long for a sweet and you *must* satisfy the craving, suck on a sourball (15 calories) or a Lifesaver (5 calories). Don't keep candy in your pockets, purse, or other convenient spots within your reach.

_____ Rearrange the refrigerator. Display in front the foods you are least likely to snack on.

_____ Chew gum (6 calories a stick) when you get the urge to eat something. Sugarless (4 calories) is recommended.

_____ Mentally rank in order the foods on your plate by calorie content. Eat the foods with the lowest calorie-content first. Perhaps you won't be so quick to consume those last few bites of high-calorie foods at the end of each meal, knowing they contain the most concentrated amount of calories.

_____ Budget calories for special occasions and holidays. This is not cheating; you're just eating calories that were allotted to you before. It *is* cheating, however, to eat more than you actually saved.

_____ Make a point to dine with friends or family. Eating alone is a common mistake of the concerned dieter. We tend to eat more balanced meals when we are with others. Conversation also slows down the fast eater, thereby giving the delayed full-feeling signal a chance to reach the brain.

_____ When possible, buy food in exactly the quantity you plan to eat. That extra ounce you may get for practically nothing extra will probably show up around your waist. Ultimately, you must decide whether that risk is outweighed by the price differentiation.

_____ Break the habit of treating or rewarding yourself with food. Reward yourself by feeling good about the calories you have saved. Reward yourself with a walk. Or ask that special person in your life for a hug.

_____ Weigh yourself only once a week. Do it at the same time, on the same scale, under the same conditions. In women, menstruation may temporarily alter the water balance, causing a weight gain of short duration.

_____ Be aware of the cues that trigger your appetite. If seeing food is the cue that sets you off, then keep food out of sight. Wrap it or store it in nonsee-through containers. Avoid temptation in so far as possible.

_____ Wrap and seal things tightly and elaborately. Tape shut the lids of jars and tins. This maneuver will cut down on odor cues. You may just decide it's too much bother to unwrap and rewrap the container for a little nibble. Each small victory is important.

DRAMATIC HINTS TO KEEP YOU INSPIRED

_____ Buy a terrific outfit in the size that will be yours when you reach your goal weight. Hang it somewhere to serve as a constant source of visual motivation.

_____ Make up signs bearing mottos such as "You can do it," "One day at a time," "Bathing suit, here I come," "A word to the wide should be sufficient"; "Win the no-belly prize," "How many did you save today?" Post them throughout the house (especially in the kitchen).

_____ Hang pictures of thin people around the house. However, on the refrigerator door, hang a picture of a grossly obese person—maybe even a picture of yourself before you began to change your life style.

_____ Place a see-through container in the front of the refrigerator. Keep it filled with raw vegetables. Print on the container "EAT-THIN SNACK PACK."

_____ Tape a sign on a full-length mirror—"You are what you eat" or "What you eat today, you'll wear tomorrow." Pause each day long enough to read the sign and look at your entire body in a relaxed state. Now suck in your stomach, hold your breath, and look again. Practice proper posture often.

_____ Keep "Summary Guidelines for Becoming THIN FROM WITHIN" (pp. 152-155) taped on the bathroom wall. Reread it each day.

Become acquainted with the following low-calorie treats:

_____ ice cubes (0 calories)—much better to suck on than hard candies

_____ radish (1 calorie)

_____ raw green pepper (10 calories)

_____ raw carrot (20 calories)

_____ broth or consommé (10-30 calories per cup)

_____ lettuce (14 calories per 3½-ounce serving)

_____ cucumber (7 calories per ½ medium, pared)

_____ popcorn with oil and salt (1 cup contains 65 calories. Cut back on oil and salt. Use no butter.)

_____ vegetable bouillon (5 calories per cube)

_____ extra-large green olive (5 calories)

_____ medium tomato (35 calories)

_____ pretzels (20 calories per 5 small sticks)

Eat a few of your meals seated in front of a mirror. Observe yourself and note in your diary your impressions about the characteristics, speed, style, and patterns of your eating habits. Seeing yourself as others see you while you're eating can bring valuable insights.

Also note in your diary your feelings while doing this exercise. What were your reactions? Did you tend to change your eating behavior? Did you eat faster? slower? more carefully?

HINTS TO INCREASE YOUR ENERGY OUTPUT

_____ Know that the risks of creeping obesity are real and that your motivation to counteract your inactivity patterns must be high. A body at rest tends to stay at rest.

_____ Learn about the benefits of increased activity, particularly in relation to a weight-reduction program.

_____ Develop a love, or at least an appreciation, for the active life. Explore the different movements of which your body is capable.

Thin From Within

_____ Engage in activities that involve the large muscles of the body, particularly the legs.

_____ Participate in activities that you enjoy. You'll be more likely to do them again and again.

_____ Don't think of increased activity as "exercise." (It may bring back unpleasant memories of physical education classes in which calisthenics may have been used as punishment.)

_____ Movement is the key to activity. Begin to move more whenever and wherever possible. Think up excuses to be more active.

_____ Stand rather than sit when appropriate—you'll use up 9 extra calories per hour. In addition, when you're standing you are more likely to move.

_____ Minimize your use of labor-saving devices. As the world enters an energy crisis, remember that excess energy (FAT) is stored within your tissues. This potential energy can best be released through movement.

_____ Walk up steps; skip the elevators and escalators.

_____ Cut your TV time by 25 to 50 percent. You won't miss it.

_____ Limit TV viewing to a specific number of hours per week. State limits here: _____.

_____ Use part of the saved time writing in your dietary diary.

_____ Invest other non-TV time in a walking program. Walking is great for burning up calories. You can do it alone or with others. You can walk to get someplace or just to take in the beauty of nature. Rain or shine, you can walk fast, slow, with long strides, on your toes, or with a bounce step. No two walks need be the same.

_____ Park your car several blocks from your destination, and walk the rest of the way.

_____ _Walk_ to the local shopping center. Think about how nice it will be not to have to look for a parking spot when you get there. If you must

54

drive, park in the farthest section of the lot.

_____ Instead of having the daily paper delivered to your house, walk briskly to the nearest newspaper stand and pick it up.

_____ Surprise friends by walking to their house.

_____ Learn to *stride*. A stride is a long step at a moderately fast pace. Striding distances can rejuvenate your spirit while you burn calories and increase your fitness level.

_____ Ask others to join you in your daily program of striding. Good company makes striding more pleasurable.

_____ Take a 10-to-15-minute brisk walk half an hour after dinner. Walking will keep your metabolic rate much higher than collapsing on the sofa in front of the television.

_____ Bike ride. If feasible, use a bike for transportation. People may stare at you, but haven't they already been giving you the stare that says, "Isn't it time you got back into things?" Besides, you're burning calories in place of gas. You're not polluting the atmosphere, and you'll be more likely to find a parking space.

_____ If you have a small lawn, use a hand-pushed lawn mower.

_____ If you golf, carry your clubs instead of pulling them on a cart. Stride after the ball between hits. The foursome behind you will appreciate your fast pace.

_____ If you enjoy calisthenics, do them to your favorite music, alternating between fast and slow tempo.

_____ Don't oversleep. Sleeping burns up fewer calories than any other activity. When you experience insomnia, get up and do some mild activity. This will tire you and increase your metabolic rate so that you will burn more calories when you do get to sleep.

_____ Beware of rainy days. Try to be active, though housebound. Movement is the key. Remember,

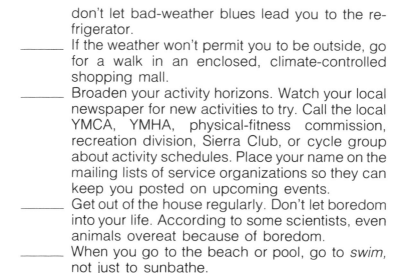

don't let bad-weather blues lead you to the re-frigerator.

_____ If the weather won't permit you to be outside, go for a walk in an enclosed, climate-controlled shopping mall.

_____ Broaden your activity horizons. Watch your local newspaper for new activities to try. Call the local YMCA, YMHA, physical-fitness commission, recreation division, Sierra Club, or cycle group about activity schedules. Place your name on the mailing lists of service organizations so they can keep you posted on upcoming events.

_____ Get out of the house regularly. Don't let boredom into your life. According to some scientists, even animals overeat because of boredom.

_____ When you go to the beach or pool, go to *swim,* not just to sunbathe.

_____ When you see a junk-food vending machine, increase your walking speed until you are well past it.

Go back and star all those items that you would feel proud to do on a regular basis.

SUMMARY OF HINTS

If you are really serious about losing weight, you should have initialed approximately 35 of the simple but sure-fire hints that decrease total caloric intake. Since activity not only burns calories but also helps to firm up sagging muscles, you should have initialed at least 15 of the hints to increase the amount and quality of your daily activity.

If you are considering a plan that does not involve a significant increase in activity, be aware of the consequences of your decision. In such a program, the only way you can lose weight (other than through surgery or drugs) is by strict caloric restriction. Your total caloric intake will need to be restricted severely (perhaps too severely) before you will make any significant progress. For example, if you choose to remain inactive and desire to lose 2 pounds per week through diet alone, you will need to eliminate 7,000 calories from your normal weekly intake, or 1,000 calories per day! If you are maintaining your present weight with 2,000 calories, a 1,000-calorie reduction would be far too drastic and might cause you to abandon the diet completely. It is difficult to have variety of foods and nutritional balance if your caloric intake is set at less than 1,200 calories per day.

One-thousand-calorie diets often leave you hungry. Hunger causes pain. Pain has discouraged many a well-intentioned dieter. Therefore, if you choose *not* to increase your activity level, it may be necessary for you to adapt yourself to mild or even severe hunger pains for the rest of your life.

If you are not willing to go hungry, some other sacrifice must be made. You must either increase your total activity level or remain at nearly your present weight. The choice is yours.

STAYING PSYCHED—WHAT TO EXPECT

There are a number of common pitfalls that the pound-shedding dieter will encounter. Knowing about them in advance should help you to avoid these traps.

1. Think—don't just react—whenever food is involved. It is easy to fall back, unconsciously, into old eating patterns.

2. Don't become too self-confident. "I've been so good for the past month, a weekend eating spree won't hurt." Not so fast! Your splurge days should be very carefully planned. Many a well-intentioned dieter, ex-smoker, or ex-drinker has stood at the same crossroad. "Cheating" before you are psychologically ready could set into motion conditioned binge-eating responses that are almost irreversible. Remember there is only a thin bottom line between "EAT" and "FAT"!

3. Weddings, birthdays, and special holidays necessitate that your food plan be flexible. In so far as possible, limit special-occasion eating to no more

than once a month. If you maintain a calorie-restricted diet and increased-activity plan, occasional prudent palate pleasing will not upset your caloric homeostasis. On days following "planned cheating," engage in extra physical activity as a reminder of the price that must be paid to maintain energy equilibrium.

4. Watch out for boredom. Keep busy—in body and mind. An idle mind and body can be a dangerous combination in a society that conditions us to eat in response to boredom. If physical activity is inappropriate at the time boredom strikes, telephone an empathetic friend and share your feelings. Or take out your diet diary and write about your feelings.

5. You are bound to experience some depression, but cultivate positive thinking. If depression is allowed to deepen, guilt may develop, and the self-defeating cycle of rejection will begin. Remember, when you're down emotionally, it won't be long until you're back up again—provided you don't stop trying.

6. Adjustment to these new eating and activity patterns of life will involve some risk—doing things about which you are unsure. Your feelings of hesitation or doubt are understandable, but unless you are willing to risk a little, not much progress can be made. Success will come in direct proportion to the amount you are willing to risk.

7. Expect compliments as you begin to lose, but accept them philosophically. Compliments that go to your head often show up around the waist.

8. As your diet and activity plan progresses past the first few weeks of weight loss, you will hit a temporary period of remission or leveling off. *Don't become discouraged!* This is to be expected. Your body is making adjustments in its water balance. Although your scale will show no significant loss of poundage, because of water retention, rest assured that calories of stored fat *are* being used for energy. Water will temporarily fill the empty spaces of the now-

shrunken fat cells. Your weight will go down within a week or so. The body will readjust its water balance and will no longer need those pouches of water— provided your salt intake is within normal limits. (Most people use more salt than is considered healthy, particularly those who regularly consume prepackaged, processed, or prepared foods.)

9. Sometimes on a calorie-restriction, activity-increase plan the scale will not reflect a weight loss, even though you *feel* and *look* lighter. Your own observations are correct, *and* your scale is accurate. You look and feel lighter in those once snug-fitting clothes because the increased activity has toned up your inactive and flabby muscles. As your muscles become stronger they will increase in density and weight. Your weight stabilization is due, in part, to a much higher percentage of protein-water concentration in your lean muscle tissues than in your more buoyant excess fat tissue. Believe your mirror. You *are* losing fat. Excess water will balance out in a week or so, and you will realize the reward for your efforts. Just remember, it's *fat* that makes you look and feel fat.

10. In your overzealousness, don't restrict your calories too severely. Consuming fewer than 1,200 calories per day may cause your body to slow down its metabolism in an attempt to conserve its stores of energy. Your body doesn't know it's on a diet. It interprets the cutback in calorie consumption as a famine and deals with the situation by slowing down the rate at which it burns food. A good way to counteract your body's tendency to conserve energy is to increase your activity. Exercise speeds up your metabolic rate and thus counterbalances the body's attempt to slow it down.

As you experience some of these pitfalls, jot down the date they happened and your thoughts and feelings in your diary. Note the situations and circumstances that you find most difficult. Keeping these feelings of frustration and discouragement locked up inside can eat away at your motivation. By writing down your feelings, you are admitting that you have them, thus preventing them from destroying your eating and activity plan.

THE I-LIKE-ME LINE

Your continued motivation will be sparked by the good feelings you have about yourself and your progress. The I-Like-Me Line is a strategy designed to focus on the positive aspects of your weight-control behavior.

We are our own worst critics. We rarely take time to reflect on and feel good about our successes for fear of becoming self-centered. But healthy acceptance of accomplishments is an essential part of your weight-control program.

Every day, write down one or more things you *did* about your food and activity plan about which you are happy. Only *actions* count, not intentions. In this way you are reinforcing and rewarding *behavior.* You may be pleased that you took a walk or used the stairs rather than the elevator. Perhaps you feel good about resisting the temptation to raid the refrigerator for a snack.

Begin now. Record something that you did today that you can be happy about.

Today I _____

_____

_____

Occasionally you will experience down days—days when you not only have no accomplishments to feel good about but also do things you regret. It is worthwhile to record such in your diary for later analysis, but don't let these thoughts destroy your motivation. At the same time that you note these discouraging feelings or experiences, write down a future I-Like-Me Line—something you plan to do later that day or early the next day that you'll feel glad about and that will outshine today's gloom.

Sharing your I-Like-Me Lines with your weight-watching friends is a good idea. Be sure to validate their Lines. Be very careful not to put down what they feel good about. You can help one another build confidence, trust, self-respect.

CRITERION FOR DETERMINING THE SUCCESS OF YOUR WEIGHT-CONTROL PLAN

You are never really cured of being overweight. The best you can ever hope for is lifetime control. You measure your success by how long you remain close to your ideal weight. Once you reach this, the plan you followed can continue in somewhat modified form as a pattern of life. Hopefully, your weight-control plan has reeducated you so that you can maintain a caloric balance without a great deal of effort. By the time you reach your ideal weight, counting calories to keep a balance between eating and activity should have become part of your personality.

Granted, you will never be able to go back to your old eating and inactivity patterns without suffering the consequences. However, after several years of continued success the urge to relapse will diminish. It's just not worth risking all you've "gained" by losing control of your caloric balance.

In fighting alcoholism, members of Alcoholics Anonymous are quick to point out that their disease may be under control, but they are still only one drink away from being a drunk. Perhaps foodaholics can measure their success the same way. You are never really cured, but after several years of successful calorie restriction and activity increase, you may consider yourself controlled. But remember—you are only a few smorgasbords away from overweight.

DEVELOPING A CALORIE CONSCIOUSNESS

Calories do count. Your caloric figures probably explain the present condition of your figure. Even if you have a poor head for figures, calorie counting can become second nature to you. You will soon develop expertise in counting two kinds of calories—those you take in and those you expend.

You should become calorie conscious in order to give yourself greater freedom and flexibility in planning your own diet. Begin to commit to memory the caloric values of the foods you normally consume.

Calorie consciousness also involves becoming familiar with your personal caloric expenditure for the wide range of physical activities you perform. You should begin to calculate your caloric needs for each day, accounting for each moment of a twenty-four-hour period. Once you have analyzed your total caloric expenditure per day, you will have a much better idea of how many calories you can safely consume.

WHAT IS A CALORIE?

An ounce is a unit measure of weight. An inch is a unit measure of length. A calorie is a unit measure of heat.

Developing a Calorie Consciousness

One calorie (sometimes referred to as a kilocalorie, or k-calorie, because it is larger than a calorie used in physics) is the amount of heat required to raise one kilogram of water one Centigrade degree.

A calorie does not measure weight; it's a measure of heat—potential heat. When speaking of body metabolism, the terms *heat, energy,* and *calories* can be used interchangeably. During the process of metabolism, the stored, potential energy is burned up, thereby producing heat. Calories are accumulated through the food we ingest. Once deposited in the body's bank account, the calorie can be spent only through heat production. There are no magical withdrawals from this bank account without the heat produced through expenditure of energy.

A calorie is not an inch, nor is it an ounce. However, since a calorie has mass, it also has measurable weight. For example, 113 calories from a carbohydrate source weigh one ounce. Since fat is the most concentrated source of energy—two and a quarter times more concentrated than carbohydrates—255 calories from a fat source weigh one ounce.

Energy stored in the form of fat is nature's way of conserving space while preserving large quantities of energy. Obviously, a pound of body fat weighs the same as a pound of carbohydrate—16 ounces, or 454 grams. The difference is in the caloric yield; the pound of fat theoretically yields 4,086 calories of heat energy, and the pound of carbohydrate yields 1,816 calories of heat energy. Actually, 4,086 calories are not stored within a pound of body fat, for approximately 12 percent of the pound is accounted for by water retention; therefore, a pound of body fat yields about 3,500 calories.

WHAT IS WATER WEIGHT?

Water has weight but no calories. One pint of water weighs one pound. Water constitutes the majority of body weight (but nothing of your body calories). Your body needs a certain amount of water to function. The body's conservation and utilization of its water supply is a very precise process. Interfering with this balance creates problems.

Weight gained through fluid retention is only temporary: Your body will eventually excrete the excess. Conversely, weight loss through excess water excretion, brought on by sweating or diuretics, is also temporary. Water balance must be maintained for physiological efficiency. A loss of water weight will show up on a scale, but the body will quickly replace it once the imbalance has been felt.

Since water contains no calories it is not burned up. Water is released from the cell as a by-product of metabolism to help stabilize body temperature. The harder you work your body, the more heat it produces. Excessive heat production causes sweating, which in turn reduces the body temperature. Sweating eliminates water weight from the body, but no fat weight is lost. This principle is important to your calorie consciousness.

For example, if you were to drink 16 fluid ounces of water, your body would store no calories, but your weight would show a temporary increase of one scale pound. If you were to drink 16 ounces of cola containing sugar worth 210 calories, the same weight gain—one pound—would show up immediately on the scale. Over time the body will utilize the fluids from both sources to balance its water supply. However, the calories from the cola drink will remain part of your total weight if not burned up. These 210 calories account for approximately 2 ounces of body weight in their carbohydrate form. If not used up by the system, these carbohydrate calories will be converted into fat calories, weighing a little less than one ounce. About 16 unused pints of cola calories would result in approximately a one pound body weight gain!

Water balance is also influenced by salt and hormones. An excess of either of these two substances will cause the body to retain more fluids than it needs. This extra weight shows up on the scale, but when appropriate adjustments are made in salt intake, excessive fluid retention generally stops.

Just prior to menstruation, many women experience a bloated feeling, which is due to an increased production of the hormone progesterone. Just as salt retains water, progesterone retains fluid. After menstruation the water balance is reinstated. Women who are using the combination estrogen-progestin birth-control pill retain this fluid for the entire cycle. The sequential birth-control pill (estrogen followed in sequence by progestin) appears to more closely simulate the normal cycle.

BEING SELECTIVE ABOUT CALORIES

If calorie counts are stored in your memory bank, perhaps they will be less likely to find their way into your body's calorie bank account.

If you consume 100 excess calories per day, you will gain about 9 to 12 pounds per year. A daily excess of 50 calories would equal a 4½-pound weight gain per year.

If you want to avoid such disaster, you will have to become adept at calorie counting. When you are thoroughly familiar with the caloric values of various foods, particularly foods within the same nutritional groups, you will find that you have much greater flexibility. Very soon you will reach the point where you can examine or plan a menu and choose portion-controlled foods that are low in calories, nutritious—*and that you like.*

You will reach the point where you are automatically making mental computations of all the calories you are consuming as you go along. Instead of restricting you, keeping a running total in your head will actually give you greater freedom. If, all during the day you are aware of how many calories you've had so far, and how many more you're still allowed, you will know whether you can have that extra cookie, glass of juice, piece of fruit. You will make choices that both please and satisfy you.

We all generally tend to overeat of foods that we like. It's a good idea to examine your favorite foods and the quantities in which you indulge in them to see whether it is worth it to eat so much of them. If you're limiting your caloric intake, the more you eat of one food, the less room there is left for other foods. The choice is yours. Make it consciously and wisely.

FAVORITE CALORIE INTAKES

In the chart provided below, list your ten favorite foods, as well as the amounts you normally consume per serving. Using your list of common foods and their calories, record the appropriate caloric content for the amount you consume.

Look over your list carefully. In view of what you now know about the nutritional value of various foods, are there any items on your list of favorites that you would now reconsider? Put a **?** next to any such item.

Are there any items that you think are excessive? Put a — next to those foods that you think you should reduce in quantity.

Which items are junk foods, providing mostly empty calories? Put **J** next to these.

Are there any items you would consider eliminating completely at this point? Mark these with an **X.**

Favorite Foods	Amount Per Serving	Calories
1.		
2.		
3.		
4.		
5.		
6.		
7.		
8.		
9.		
10.		

Developing a Calorie Consciousness

Choose the food that is your least favorite and figure out how many calories you would save in a month if you eliminated it completely. Multiply the calories per serving by how many times you would normally have eaten this food in a month.

Food: _____

_____ Calories

x 31 days = _____ calories per month.

CALORIE COUNTING

Calorie counting will eventually become automatic to you. At first it is a cumbersome procedure that requires memorization and much repetition for reinforcement. However, just as with memorizing the keys on the typewriter or piano, eventually the task becomes a skill, taken over by the autonomic nervous system. The following drill will help familiarize you with the caloric content of selected foods in different groups.

PLAYING THE CALORIE GAME

In the chart below, the foods are listed in alphabetical order within each category. Your task is to place the foods in sequence according to their caloric content. Rank as number one the food you think is highest in calories in that group; then guesstimate the number of calories for that food.

Category	Food		Rank	Estimated Calories	Actual Calories
Drinks	Cola Skim milk Whole milk	8 oz. 8 oz. 8 oz.			
Vege-tables	Celery stalks Potato Potato chips	10 large 1 med. boiled 9 me- dium			

Thin From Within

Category	Food		Rank	Estimated Calories	Actual Calories
Snacks	Chocolate kisses Peanuts, salted Pizza, cheese Raisins	7 1 oz. ⅛ of 14″ pie 1 oz.			
Ice Cream	Chocolate Orange ice Orange sherbet Strawberry Vanilla	1/6 qt. 1/6 qt. 1/6 qt. 1/6 qt. 1/6 qt.			
Fruits	Apple Banana Navel orange Peach Pear	1 me- dium 6 inch 1 large 4 oz. 1 me- dium			
Candy	Caramels Chocolate bar w. almonds Gumdrops Jellybeans Marshmallows	3 1 oz. 20 10 4 large			
Fruit Juice	Grapefruit juice, fresh Grape juice Lime, fresh Orange juice Tomato juice	1 cup (8 oz.) 1 cup 1 1 cup 1 cup			

Drinks: 105, 90, 160
Vegetables: 80, 76, 97
Snacks: 152, 162, 185, 80
Ice Cream: 200, 96, 177, 169, 193
Fruits: 70, 85, 65, 35, 100
Candy: 115, 150, 100, 105, 90
Fruit juice: 95, 135, 60, 110, 50

Developing a Calorie Consciousness

The following charts should familiarize you with the wide variations in calorie content that exist within groups of apparently similar foods. Differences come from the foods themselves, as well as from the form of preparation. Observe how the fat content of food (particularly fried forms) inflates the calorie content.

Different Caloric Values of Potatoes, Depending on Method of Preparation (All values are for 100-gm. [3½ oz.] servings)	
Type of Preparation	Calories
Raw white	76
Boiled, peeled	65
Boiled in skin	76
Baked, peeled after baking	93
Mashed, milk added	65-78
Mashed, milk and margarine added	94-120
French fried, frozen	220
French fried, fresh	274
Hashbrowns	229
Potato sticks	300
Potato chips, crisp	568

Different Caloric Values of Various Forms of Milk (All values are for 8 oz. servings)	
Type	Calories
Regular milk	
3.5% butterfat	160
2% butterfat	140
1% butterfat	115
Skim milk	90-98
Buttermilk	98
Chocolate-flavored milk	212
Half-and-half	325
Eggnog	474

Thin From Within

Different Caloric Values of Breads	
(All values are for 1-slice servings)	
Type	Calories
Boston brown	100
Cracked wheat	65
French	63
Gluten	35
Italian	62
Profile	52
Protein	45
Pumpernickel	77
Raisin	62
Rye, light	53
Vienna	63
White	64
Whole wheat	57

Different Caloric Values of Common Snack Foods		
Type	Approximate Measure	Calories
Beverages		
Carbonated, cola type	6 oz.	70
Chocolate milk (made with skim milk)	1 cup	190
Cocoa	1 cup	235
Malted milk	1½ cups	420
Vanilla-ice-cream soda	1½ cups	260

Different Caloric Values of Common Snack Foods		
Type	Approximate Measure	Calories
Cake		
Angel food	2″ sector	110
Cream puff, custard filling	1 average	245
Cupcake, chocolate, iced	1	185
Doughnut, jelly	1 average	225
Doughnut, plain	1 average	125
Doughnut, raised	1 average	120
Fruitcake	2 x 2 x 1½″	115
Candy		
Butterscotch	3 pieces	60
Candy bar, plain	1	295
Chocolate-coated creams	2 average	130
Fudge	1 piece	115
Peanut brittle	1 oz.	125
Popcorn (with oil)	1 cup	65
Cheese		
Camembert	1 oz.	85
Cheddar	1 oz.	105
Cream	1 oz.	105
Swiss (domestic)	1 oz.	105
Cookies		
Brownie	2 x 2 x ¾″	140
Plain assorted	3 inch	120
Crackers		
Cheese	5	85
Graham	2 medium	55
Rye	2	45
Saltines	4	70

Different Caloric Values of Common Snack Foods		
Type	Approximate Measure	Calories
Nuts		
Mixed, shelled	8-12	95
Peanut butter	1 Tbs.	95
Peanuts, shelled, roasted	1 cup	840
Pie		
Apple	4″ sector	345
Cherry	4″ sector	355
Custard	4″ sector	280
Lemon meringue	4″ sector	305
Mince	4″ sector	365
Pumpkin	4″ sector	275
Sandwiches		
Cheese	1	225
Egg salad	1	280
Lettuce and tomato	1	135
Peanut butter	1	330
Soups, commercial canned		
Cream of celery	1 cup	160
Cream of mushroom	1 cup	135
Cream of potato	1 cup	150
Onion	1 cup	57
Tomato	1 cup	90
Split pea	1 cup	150
Vegetable bouillon	1 cup	8
Vegetarian vegetable	1 cup	76

Different Caloric Values of Common Snack Foods		
Type	Approximate Measure	Calories
Broccoli	1 stalk	32
Carrot	1 medium	20
Celery	1 stalk	5
Green pepper	1 medium	10
Jams, jellies, marmalades, preserves	1 Tbs.	55
Sherbet	½ cup	120
Syrup	¼ cup	240
Waffle	4½x5½x½"	210

FOOD-ACTIVITY CALORIC EQUIVALENTS

Food contains calories. Activity uses calories. Excessive eating will take its toll unless something is done to counter it. *Quid pro quo* ("Something in exchange for something") should become part of your unconscious caloric-balancing act. "If I do such and such at the table, then I need to do so and so as an activity to balance it out." For every excess calorie you eat, there must be a counterbalancing activity period. If not, you will surely gain weight.

How long would it take to walk off a large apple? Run off a doughnut? Sleep off a chocolate layer cake? How long would it take to work off a milkshake by walking? by golfing? by sitting? running? swimming?

The following chart will give you a relative idea of how many minutes it would take to work off various food items through certain activities. For example, in fifteen minutes, you could walk off a boiled egg, bicycle off a glass of orange juice, or swim off a helping of jelly beans. The same calories *could* be burned up if you do nothing but sit around; however, it would take almost two hours!

Activity Equivalents of Various Foods *

FOOD	Calories/Minute	Apple	Banana	Beans, green	Bread and butter	Cake
Running	19.4	5	5	1	4	18
Walking Up Stairs or Hills	18.3	6	5	1	4	19
Swimming	11.0	9	8	2	7	32
Playing Handball	10.2	10	9	3	8	35
Playing Tennis	7.1	14	12	4	11	50
Jogging	10.0	10	9	3	8	36
Striding 4.5 mph	7.0	14	13	4	11	51
Walking 3.5 mph	5.2	19	17	5	15	68
Cycling 10 mph	8.0	13	11	3	10	45
Cycling 5.5 mph	4.5	22	20	6	17	79
Golfing	5.0	20	18	5	16	71
Bowling	4.4	23	20	6	18	81
Ironing	4.2	24	21	6	19	85
Making Beds	3.9	26	23	7	20	91
Preparing Meals	3.3	31	27	8	24	108
Driving a Car	2.8	36	31	10	28	127
Typing or Playing Piano	2.5	40	35	11	31	142
Standing or Sitting and Writing	1.9	53	46	14	41	187
Reclining	1.4	72	63	19	56	254
Sleeping	1.0	101	88	27	78	356
CALORIES		101	88	27	78	356
QUANTITY		1 lg.	1 sm.	1 cup	1 sl. pat	1 wdg.

Activity Equivalents of Various Foods

FOOD	Running	Walking Up Stairs or Hills	Swimming	Playing Handball	Playing Tennis	Jogging	Striding 4.5 mph	Walking 3.5 mph	Cycling 10 mph	Cycling 5.5 mph	Golfing	Bowling	Ironing	Making Beds	Preparing Meals	Driving a Car	Typing or Playing Piano	Standing or Sitting and Writing	Reclining	Sleeping	CALORIES	QUANTITY
Calories/Minute	19.4	18.3	11.0	10.2	7.1	10.0	7.0	5.2	8.0	4.5	5.0	4.4	4.2	3.9	3.3	2.8	2.5	1.9	1.4	1.0		
Candy, caramel	6	6	11	12	17	12	17	23	15	26	24	27	28	30	36	42	47	62	84	118	118	1 oz.
Candy, chocolate fudge	6	6	11	12	17	12	17	23	15	26	24	27	28	30	36	42	47	62	84	118	118	1¼"
Candy, hard, all flavors	6	6	10	11	15	11	16	21	14	24	22	25	26	28	33	39	44	58	79	110	110	1 oz.
Candy, Hershey bar	11	11	19	20	29	21	30	40	26	46	42	48	50	54	63	75	84	110	149	209	209	1⅜ oz.
Candy, jelly beans	3	4	6	6	9	7	9	13	8	15	13	15	16	17	20	24	26	35	47	66	66	10
Carrot, raw	2	2	4	4	6	4	6	8	5	9	8	10	10	11	13	15	17	22	30	42	42	3 oz.

Activity Equivalents of Various Foods

FOOD	Calories/Minute →	QUANTITY	CALORIES	Running 19.4	Walking Up Stairs or Hills 18.3	Swimming 11.0	Playing Handball 10.2	Playing Tennis 7.1	Jogging 10.0	Striding 4.5 mph 7.0	Walking 3.5 mph 5.2	Cycling 10 mph 8.0	Cycling 5.5 mph 4.5	Golfing 5.0	Bowling 4.4	Ironing 4.2	Making Beds 3.9	Preparing Meals 3.3	Driving a Car 2.8	Typing or Playing Piano 2.5	Standing or Sitting and Writing 1.9	Reclining 1.4	Sleeping 1.0
Cheese, cheddar		1 oz.	111	6	6	10	11	16	11	16	21	14	25	22	25	26	28	34	40	44	58	79	111
Cheese, cottage		1 Tbs.	27	1	1	2	3	4	3	4	5	3	6	5	6	6	7	8	10	11	14	19	27
Cookies, plain		148/lb.	15	1	1	1	1	2	2	2	3	2	3	3	3	4	4	5	5	6	8	11	15
Cookie, chocolate chip		1 avg.	51	3	3	5	5	7	5	7	10	6	11	10	12	12	13	15	18	20	27	36	51
Doughnut		1 avg.	151	8	8	14	15	21	15	22	29	19	34	30	34	36	39	46	54	60	79	108	151

Activity Equivalents of Various Foods

FOOD	QUANTITY	CALORIES	Sleeping	Reclining	Standing or Sitting and Writing	Typing or Playing Piano	Driving a Car	Preparing Meals	Making Beds	Ironing	Bowling	Golfing	Cycling 5.5 mph	Cycling 10 mph	Walking 3.5 mph	Striding 4.5 mph	Jogging	Playing Tennis	Playing Handball	Swimming	Walking Up Stairs or Hills	Running
Calories/Minute			1.0	1.4	1.9	2.5	2.8	3.3	3.9	4.2	4.4	5.0	4.5	8.0	5.2	7.0	10.0	7.1	10.2	11.0	18.3	19.4
Egg, boiled	1	77	77	55	41	31	28	23	20	18	18	15	17	10	15	11	8	11	8	7	4	4
Egg, fried	1	110	110	79	58	44	39	33	28	26	25	22	24	14	21	16	11	15	11	10	6	6
French dressing	1 Tbs.	59	59	42	31	24	21	18	15	14	13	12	13	7	11	8	6	8	6	5	3	3
Ice cream	1/6 qt.	193	193	138	102	77	69	58	49	46	44	39	43	24	37	28	19	27	19	18	11	10
Ice-cream soda	1 glass	255	255	182	134	102	91	77	65	61	58	51	57	32	49	36	26	36	25	23	14	13

Activity Equivalents of Various Foods

FOOD	Running (19.4)	Walking Up Stairs or Hills (18.3)	Swimming (11.0)	Playing Handball (10.2)	Playing Tennis (7.1)	Jogging (10.0)	Striding 4.5 mph (7.0)	Walking 3.5 mph (5.2)	Cycling 10 mph (8.0)	Cycling 5.5 mph (4.5)	Golfing (5.0)	Bowling (4.4)	Ironing (4.2)	Making Beds (3.9)	Preparing Meals (3.3)	Driving a Car (2.8)	Typing or Playing Piano (2.5)	Standing or Sitting and Writing (1.9)	Reclining (1.4)	Sleeping (1.0)	CALORIES	QUANTITY
Jello with cream	6	6	11	11	16	12	17	23	15	26	23	27	28	30	35	42	47	62	84	117	117	½ cup
Mayonnaise	5	5	8	9	13	9	13	18	12	20	18	21	22	24	28	33	37	48	66	92	92	1 Tbs.
Milk, skim	4	4	7	8	11	8	12	16	10	18	16	18	19	21	25	29	32	43	58	81	81	1 glass
Milk, whole	9	9	15	16	23	17	24	32	21	37	33	38	40	43	50	59	66	87	119	166	166	1 glass
Milkshake	22	23	38	41	59	42	60	81	53	94	84	96	100	108	128	150	168	222	301	421	421	12 oz.
Milkshake, malted	26	27	46	49	71	50	72	97	63	112	100	114	120	129	152	179	201	264	359	502	502	12 oz.

Activity Equivalents of Various Foods

FOOD	Calories/Minute	Orange	Orange juice	Pancake with syrup	Peach	Peas, green	Pie, apple
QUANTITY		1 med.	8 oz.	1	1 med.	½ cup	⅙ pie
CALORIES		68	120	124	46	56	377
Running	19.4	4	6	6	2	3	19
Walking Up Stairs or Hills	18.3	4	7	7	3	3	21
Swimming	11.0	6	11	11	4	5	34
Playing Handball	10.2	7	12	12	5	5	37
Playing Tennis	7.1	10	17	17	6	8	53
Jogging	10.0	7	12	12	5	6	38
Striding 4.5 mph	7.0	10	17	18	7	8	54
Walking 3.5 mph	5.2	13	23	24	9	11	73
Cycling 10 mph	8.0	9	15	16	6	7	47
Cycling 5.5 mph	4.5	15	27	28	10	12	84
Golfing	5.0	14	24	25	9	11	75
Bowling	4.4	15	27	28	10	13	86
Ironing	4.2	16	29	30	11	13	90
Making Beds	3.9	17	31	32	12	14	97
Preparing Meals	3.3	21	36	38	14	17	114
Driving a Car	2.8	24	43	44	16	20	135
Typing or Playing Piano	2.5	27	48	50	18	22	151
Standing or Sitting and Writing	1.9	36	63	65	24	29	198
Reclining	1.4	49	86	89	33	40	269
Sleeping	1.0	68	120	124	46	56	377

Activity Equivalents of Various Foods

FOOD	QUANTITY	CALORIES	Running 19.4	Walking Up Stairs or Hills 18.3	Swimming 11.0	Playing Handball 10.2	Playing Tennis 7.1	Jogging 10.0	Striding 4.5 mph 7.0	Walking 3.5 mph 5.2	Cycling 10 mph 8.0	Cycling 5.5 mph 4.5	Golfing 5.0	Bowling 4.4	Ironing 4.2	Making Beds 3.9	Preparing Meals 3.3	Driving a Car 2.8	Typing or Playing Piano 2.5	Standing or Sitting and Writing 1.9	Reclining 1.4	Sleeping 1.0
Calories/Minute																					
Pie, raisin	1/6 pie	437	23	24	40	43	62	44	62	84	55	97	87	99	104	112	132	156	175	230	312	437
Pizza, cheese	1/8 pie	180	9	10	16	18	25	18	26	35	23	40	36	41	43	46	55	64	72	95	129	180
Potato chips	1 svg.	108	6	6	10	11	15	11	15	21	14	24	22	25	26	28	33	39	43	57	77	108
Sherbet	1/6 qt.	177	9	10	16	17	25	18	25	34	22	39	35	40	42	45	54	63	71	93	126	177
Spaghetti with tomato sauce	1 cup	179	20	22	36	18	56	18	57	76	50	88	79	90	94	102	120	141	158	208	283	179
Strawberry shortcake, including berries and cream	5 oz.	400	21	22	36	39	56	40	57	77	50	89	80	91	95	103	121	143	160	211	286	400

VARIATIONS WITHIN FOOD GROUPS

Variety is the spice of life; we do get tired of eating the same foods all the time. Often we shift from one food item to another within the same group, assuming that the caloric value is more or less the same. This may not turn out to be so at all.

If a person does tend to eat high-calorie foods, becoming more active will help to keep the weight under control. Plan to refer to the Activity Equivalents of Various Foods Chart often.

In the white space remaining on pages 74 to 80, jot down some of your feelings, impressions, and conclusions regarding the relationship of activity, calorie intake, and diet.

---

* Adapted and expanded by Helen Derwin (student, Towson State University) from a chart in Frank Konishi's "Calorie Equivalents of Activity," *Journal of the American Dietetic Association,* March, 1965, p. 187.

DETERMINING YOUR IDEAL WEIGHT

HEIGHT-WEIGHT BODY-FRAME CHARTS

Insurance companies are in the business of life. They know that the longer you live, the longer you pay policy premiums. Therefore, it is to the companies' advantage to keep you alive as long as possible. The height-weight body-frame charts that these companies have published reflect their statistical research findings: The shorter the waist line, the longer the life. Some authorities feel that standard height-weight body-frame charts, such as those on page 83 may be approximately 4 to 10 pounds *under* what a person's ideal weight may really be. This is a good point to keep in mind when perusing these charts; otherwise, they may be hazardous to your mental health.

Useful as these charts could be in giving a general idea of suitable weight, they are unfortunately not accompanied by instructions for determining whether you have a large, medium, or small frame. Consequently, most persons incorrectly arrive at a conclusion such as this: "Well, I'm such and such a height, and my present weight is within the range of pounds listed under 'Large

Desirable Weights for Men[1]
Men of Ages 25 and Over

Weight in Pounds According to Frame (in Indoor Clothing)			
HEIGHT (with shoes on) 1-inch heels Feet Inches	SMALL FRAME	MEDIUM FRAME	LARGE FRAME
5 2	112-120	118-129	126-141
5 3	115-123	121-133	129-144
5 4	118 126	124-136	132-148
5 5	121-129	127-139	135-152
5 6	124-133	130-143	138-156
5 7	128-137	134-147	142-161
5 8	132-141	138-152	147-166
5 9	136-145	142 156	151-170
5 10	140-150	146-160	155-174
5 11	144-154	150-165	159-179
6 0	148-158	154-170	164-184
6 1	152-162	158-175	168-189
6 2	156-167	162-180	173-194

Desirable Weights for Women[1]
Women of Ages 25 and Over

Weight in Pounds According to Frame (in Indoor Clothing)			
HEIGHT (with shoes on) 2-inch heels Feet Inches	SMALL FRAME	MEDIUM FRAME	LARGE FRAME
4 10	92- 98	96-107	104-119
4 11	94-101	98-110	106-122
5 0	96-104	101-113	109-125
5 1	99-107	104-116	112-128
5 2	102-110	107-119	115-131
5 3	105-113	110-122	118-134
5 4	108-116	113-126	121-138
5 5	111-119	116-130	125-142
5 6	114-123	120-135	129-146
5 7	118-127	124-139	133-150
5 8	122-131	128-143	137-154
5 9	126-135	132-147	141-158
5 10	130-140	136-151	145-163

Frame'; therefore, I must have a large frame."

Here are two simple ways by which you can fairly accurately determine your frame size:

1. Circle your wrist with your index finger and thumb. Be sure to use your index finger and not your middle finger. Try as hard as possible to have your thumb and index finger meet or overlap. If they will not meet at all, you have a large frame; if they just barely touch or overlap, you have a medium frame; if your thumb and index finger overlap, you have a small frame.

2. If you are a woman and the circumference of your wrist is 6 inches or less, you have a small frame; if it is between 6 and 6½ inches, your frame is medium; if it is greater than 6½ inches, your frame is large.

    If you are a man, your frame is small if your wrist circumference is less than 6 inches; medium if it is between 6 and 7 inches; and large if it is greater than 7 inches.

These methods of determining frame size are based on average measurements of thousands of people. They are accurate for 95 in 100 persons. Obviously, there may be special individual differences (such as formerly broken wrists or extremely short fingers) that would make for exceptions.

Most people are surprised to find out they are actually one frame size smaller than they thought. Perhaps that's "wristful" thinking!

MIRROR TEST

The mirror test is a search for visible fat, bulges, rolls, spare tires, et cetera. Standing nude in front of a full-length mirror, carefully inspect your body for observable traces of excessive fat. If you look fat in front of a looking glass, you probably are fat. By such an inspection, you can easily discern where you need to reduce, as well as where you need to firm up. One caution: Be sure to stand back at least six feet from the mirror. If you stand too close there will be some optical distortion, making you look fatter than you really are.

ANSWER THESE QUESTIONS IN YOUR DIARY

How do you feel about the way you look in the mirror? Can you see yourself objectively? Or are you viewing yourself through a distorted carnival fun house mirror? Many dieters have been overweight for so long that their fat image is imbedded in their brain. Even after they do begin to lose weight, they see their old selves whenever they stand before the looking glass.

If the mirror, viewed objectively, says you're fat, don't kid yourself—you're fat. But be just as realistic in your self-appraisal when the mirror says you're making progress. It may take considerable time looking at and studying yourself in front of a mirror, but eventually you will change your self-image and feel good about yourself.

THE "CUBED MIRROR" TEST

This test involves other people and takes into consideration not only the physical aspects of one's ideal weight but also the social aspects. Your ideal weight is that at which you—

Feel, look, and act best
1. To yourself.
2. To members of the same sex.
3. To members of the opposite sex.

After you have used the mirror test to make your own judgment about your ideal weight, solicit the opinions of several people of both sexes. Remember to tell them to consider not only how you look to them but also how you feel and act, as they see it.

Sometimes we look OK at a particular weight and yet feel heavy. Friends of the same sex will probably give you their honest opinions. However, remember that most women believe it is impossible to be too thin. This high-fashion thinness is not necessarily what most males desire. Among certain African tribes, steatopygia—having a big rump—is highly prized. The woman with the largest derriere, which is often shaped with baling wire, is considered the most beautiful in the tribe. Don't take off for Africa. Somewhere in between scrawniness and steatopygia there exists a realistic balance.

INTERPRETING OVERWEIGHT

No one method of determining your ideal weight is so accurate that it should be taken as the final word. Using certain criteria, many people whose weight falls within normal limits could be considered overweight, or even obese, at different points in their lives. Most well-trained athletes are overweight according to the criteria of height-weight body-frame charts. Therefore, the Public Health Service has cautioned:

"It cannot be overstressed that assigning a label of obese to any one person or group of persons should come only after a comprehensive assessment of all pertinent factors. The sex of the subject, age, body type, and state of health, along with specific measurements such as skinfold thickness, must be considered in determining if a person is obese. Comparing any individual or group in terms of their heights and weights with a given set of averages or standards does not give adequate information on which to assess obesity since such comparisons imply weight not fatness."[2]

THE PINCH TEST, OR SKINFOLD MEASUREMENT

Approximately 50 percent of all body fat is located just under the skin. The subcutaneous (under the skin) fat can be measured by pinching the skin with thumb and forefinger, and gently pulling the skin and fat away from the underlying muscle tissue. An ideal fat pinch (in a warm climate) would be between one quarter and one half of an inch. Average, or normal, fat measurements (skinfolds) would range between one half and three fourths of an inch. If the pinch test finds you holding more than an inch, you have more body fat than is considered ideal.

Determining Your Ideal Weight

It's quite possible to be overfat and not be overweight. Your weight can be great, but "fat's where it's at"! The scale weighs bone, muscle, and water, as well as fat. You can rapidly change your body weight by starvation, medication, or dehydration. But it takes a change in caloric balance—for a week or more—to significantly change your fat measurements. In other words, you can't cheat on the skinfold test as you can on the scale.

Apply the pinch test to three areas to determine your level of fatness:

1. Pinch the back of the relaxed arm, midway between the elbow and the shoulder. (This site is known as the triceps area.) Sometimes it's easier to ask another person to make the measurement for you.

   The triceps skinfold generally reveals the number of excess calories that you have eaten and stored. If the fat is firm and tight, you've probably been overfat for years, perhaps even since childhood. If the fat is loose and flabby, it generally indicates that you are in a negative caloric state; i.e., you are losing fat. Occasionally persons inherit the tendency to have fat arms. These can run in families, but if the other test sites are also overfat—don't blame your parents.

2. The top of the hip bone (suprailiac area) is another site to pinch for excess fat. Pinch and pull the skin tissue just above the bones. If you can pinch an inch or more you're overfat. (Be careful not to pinch too high up or too far back from the hip.)

   This site, also called the iliac crest, generally reveals the amount of physical activity that you do, particularly that involving the legs. Throughout the body, fat is somewhat evenly distributed, but if you are very active or inactive the hip skinfold measurement will reveal that. Low hip fat indicates an active life style. If your hip fat exceeds an inch it generally means that you lead an inactive life style.

Have you been watching too much television? Perhaps it's time to begin that walking program. A consistent half-hour-a-day walk will prove effective in controlling hip fat. Allow six to eight weeks and you'll be able to measure the difference.

3. The stomach (abdominal) area is a common site for excess fat accumulation in the post-30-year-old. Pinch for an inch of fat alongside of the navel.

The higher the fat accumulation at this site, the more sitting the individual does (in addition to consuming excess calories). The characteristic "middle-America bulge" can even happen to individuals who exercise for half an hour each day, particularly if they are sedentary for the other twenty-three and one-half hours!

Look around. Sagging abdomens are everywhere. Even sporty, active people may have that paunchy, pouchy appearance. It is not unusual to see middle-America bulge on strong-armed construction workers. In fact, some males actually take pride in their "beer bellies," claiming "good living" as the cause.

It's the author's belief that the Creator did not intend our body temples to be overrun with caloric excesses or deprived of physical activity. Our bodies are on loan from God. We're just stewards—tenants—of our physical houses. Rental of these homes is free, provided we maintain them with tender, loving care. Perhaps the Great Lessor allows for the early termination of the unhealthy tenant.

Less sitting, fewer calories, and more walking will help reduce stomach fat. The abdominal muscles under the fat can be strengthened by doing bent-leg sit-ups. This style sit-up will prevent that saggy stomach feeling, can help you lose inches from around the waist, and give some protection against low back pain. All that for just one minute of effort three times a week!

SUMMARY OF THE PINCH TEST

Record the approximate pinch results for the three measurement sites:

_____ triceps

_____ suprailiac

_____ abdominal

_____ TOTAL approximate pinch-inches

If you have a total of 2½ inches or more, you are overfat. Furthermore, a pinch of more than an inch in at least one site also indicates overfatness. Yes, even if you are of nearly normal weight and don't look fat, perhaps you had better begin a fat-reduction plan.

Excess fat deposits can affect your performance levels and detract from your health. (However, if you live in a very cold climate some excess fat tissue is helpful as insulation and protection from the cold.)

SCIENTIFIC SKINFOLD MEASUREMENTS

A more accurate assessment of your fat tissue can be made with a special instrument called a skinfold caliper. Metal skinfold calipers are very expensive. Recently a few companies have produced accurate, low-cost plastic calipers.

Two of these are:
Fat-O-Meter
2442 Irving Park Road
Chicago, Ill. 60618

Fat Control, Inc.
P.O. Box 101117
Towson, Maryland 21204

BODY IMAGE VERSUS BODY REALITY

What you see is not always what you are. As mentioned before, overweight individuals often view themselves as if through distorted glasses. This distortion can work in several ways. Sometimes the overweight person may see himself as heavier than he really is. When he looks into a mirror, he sees a bigger than actual abdomen, larger buttocks, and huge thighs. This self-image is difficult to shake even if the person's weight actually decreases markedly.

Those with realistic body concepts tend to have the greatest success in their weight-control programs, because dieters must continually reassess their body image as they lose weight.

Nothing could be more devastating to an individual whose scale says he has lost a significant amount of weight than looking into the mirror and seeing his old, pudgy self. This person can see himself only as fat. Yet most weight-control plans fail to consider this important psychological mechanism of self-perception.

Few successful dieters actually see themselves as thin, particularly when they first reach their ideal weight. Only after months of living a thin life does the successful dieter begin to feel good about himself. Once he has reached his ideal weight, the individual must take time to enjoy himself and rediscover his own beauty. He must study himself in front of a mirror, and not be afraid to respect himself.

---

[1] Courtesy of the Metropolitan Life Insurance Company, New York, N.Y.
[2] U.S. Public Health Service. *Obesity and Health* (Washington, D.C.: U.S. Government Printing Office, no date), p. 2.

YOU ARE WHAT YOU EAT

If people really were what they ate, then they might look like "hamburgerfrenchfrypotatochipicecreamhot-dogchocolatecakepopcornpizzapickle" people.

However, thanks to our genetic code, our bodies utilize the nutrients from these various foodstuffs, and rebuild them according to their DNA blueprints. Bio-chemically speaking, then, what you eat today will walk and talk tomorrow.

Your body requires approximately fifty-six different nutrients. These must be consumed on a regular basis if your system is to function efficiently and comfortably.

Even though you're on a diet, you can still consume all of these necessary nutrients without too much hassle. And if you're among the many dieters who are interested in their appearance, paying attention to nutrients will pay off. Disregarding nutritional requirements works *against* your appearance in subtle ways. A diet devoid of fresh fruits and vegetables, for example, may cost you the clear skin, bright eyes, and that healthy hair you've always liked.

So, while you're cutting down on the quantity of food you eat, make sure that what you do eat contains adequate nutrients. Overfed people are generally over-weight. But overweight people can actually be mal-nourished, because of the low-nutrient foods they choose to consume. Cut down on those fats and sugars!

THE $100,000 HABIT

If you live 70 years you will probably have eaten more than 75,000 meals! And that doesn't include parties, snacks, and nibbles! At today's skyrocketing market prices, it is almost impossible to prepare a meal for less than one dollar per person. Therefore, the bottom line on a lifetime meal ticket easily exceeds $100,000! Further-more, if you are the "average American" you purchase almost every other meal outside of the home. Have you tried lately to purchase a nutritiously adequate meal in a restaurant for a little over a dollar?

One would think that the amount of time and money we invest in eating would proportionately reflect our knowledge and practices about nutrition. On the con-trary, dietary behavior often reveals only the depth of ignorance.

Most people are not in the habit of talking about the nutritional aspects of food. Perhaps this is because eating is one of the things most people would rather do than talk about. Just as a child picks up negative, nonverbal information about sexuality, so does he un-consciously learn about nutrition, absorbing the misin-formation and misconceptions of his elders. It seems ironic that in our enlightened society children grow up with a high degree of ignorance in these two important areas.

These children will become adults and, eventually, parents. Unless considerable amounts of time and effort are invested to improve their nutritional knowledge, the cycle of ignorance will be perpetuated. The misconcep-tions that have been passed down have produced a generation of Americans whose nutritional practices blatantly oppose what is known to be true and healthful.

Nutritional ignorance is not limited to any particular

economic or ethnic group. Most people, whatever their status, suffer from intellectual retardation regarding nutrition, having an almost total lack of any functional knowledge. Surprising as it may seem, the large majority of people know scarcely more about nutrition as fullgrown adults than they did as infants.

It would seem logical that, since we spend so much time, energy, and money on eating, the prudent individual would be willing to devote an appropriate number of hours learning about nutrition. If this were done, the basic level of knowledge accumulated could make a significant contribution to his health for the rest of his life.

Any interested individual can inform himself through a personally motivated reading program or by taking an adult-education course. But, ideally, nutrition information should be taught as part of a sound health-education program, so that most people would be exposed to it during their earlier years of formal education.

DIETARY ANALYSIS/SEARCH

On the following chart, begin to keep a record of all the foods that you consume for the next three to seven days. After you have a representative sample of your eating patterns and meals, then you are ready for trouble-shooting.

Go through the listing for each meal, and wherever fats or sugars have been used, circle those items in red. (Red is a "stop" color. The sooner you stop the fat/sugar practices, the sooner you'll be in control of your eating habits.)

Fats are hidden in many of our foods. By not eating meats, the vegetarian eliminates about one third to one half of the fats normally consumed by the meat eater. But beware of fried foods, creamed foods, dressings, gravies, butter, margarine, et cetera.

Sugar is not always easy to spot. It has been added to many of the foods that we purchase. Don't be fooled by the use of brown sugar, honey, dextrose, glucose, or molasses. They are all forms of sweeteners.

Thin From Within

Whatever your number of red circles on your week's dietary search, try to cut back the number and/or serving sizes, of these foods by at least one half. For most overweight persons, fats and sugars cause 90 percent of their problem.

Day of Week & Date	Foods Consumed			Daily Food Intake		
	Breakfast	Amt.	Lunch	Amt.	Dinner	Amt.	Snacks	Amt.

FOODS I LOVE MOST TO EAT AND DRINK

On the following chart, list your eight favorite foods. Be sure to include those that you may eat only on special occasions, such as birthdays, or during certain seasons of the year. Enter the date on which you last had each food.

Put checks in the appropriate columns, using the following coding:

A Food you prefer to eat or drink when alone

⊦ Relatively high in nutrients

— High in calories and low in nutrients—"junk foods"

＊ Low in calories

Food that you eat too much of and/or too often

¢ Costs less than 50 cents a portion

$ Costs more than $2 a portion

5 Would not have been on your list 5 years ago

☺ Food that you feel happy just thinking about

! Food you plan to cut out of your life style

TV Food you eat while watching TV

: Food you plan to eat smaller portions of.

Favorite Foods	Date	A	+	−	*	#	¢	$	5	☺	!	TV	:
1.													
2.													
3.													
4.													
5.													
6.													
7.													
8.													

Objectively study the coding you have checked, just as a scientist would interpret data. Look for patterns you may not have been aware of before. For example, are the junk foods also the foods you eat when you're alone in front of the television? You will probably be amazed at the eating patterns you discover.

1. What did the eight-favorite-foods exercise reveal to you about your food selection?

2. What, if anything, do you plan to *do* about your diet as a result of this exercise?

3. Go back and circle in red the foods that are high in fats and/or sugars. What do you plan to do to regulate these foods in your life?

KNOW YOUR "FEED" LIMITS

This strategy teaches you to set realistic and reasonable limits to your food-health practices. It is designed to allow you to respond in amount or serving size as to what is enough, what is too much, and what is not enough. For those foods that are your problem foods, circle the "ENOUGH" limit in red. That should be your cue to STOP! Tomorrow is another day, and once your allotment for the day or week is gone—it's gone. By setting realistic and reasonable "feed" limits you give yourself permission to eat foods that on restrictive diets are strictly forbidden.

Obviously, if you can't eat just one without being set off on a binge, then maybe one for you would be too much. In the blank item spaces write in additional foods that are your potential binge foods.

The quibble column is for your clarification and additional information. Use it for whatever you deem appropriate. Be sure to write a summary statement about this activity somewhere in your diary.

KNOW YOUR LIMITS*

ITEM	ENOUGH	TOO MUCH	NOT ENOUGH	QUIBBLE COLUMN
1. Candy				
2. Donuts/pastry				
3. Butter/margarine				
4. Ice cream				
5. Dessert (_____)				
6. Fried foods				
8. Reading about weight control				
9. Dietary diary writing				
10. Sugar				
11. Whole-grain foods				
12. Milk/cheese				
13.				
14.				

TO THINK ABOUT AND TO WRITE ABOUT

1. Make a general statement about your behavior and/or insight from the above activity.

_____

_____

2. What behavior changes do you plan to make in the near future to improve your dietary habits?
By when? _____

_____   _____
_____
     your signature   *today's date*

* Modified from a values realization workshop by Dr. Sid Simon.

A LITTLE NUTRITION WITH YOUR WEIGHT CONTROL, PLEASE!

Too many of today's popular weight-control schemes are concerned only with the shedding of pounds. If you plan to be on a moderately reduced-calorie-intake plan for longer than a few weeks, you should be aware of the nutritional value of your weight-control plan.

An alcoholic can try to avoid booze completely. A heroin addict can attempt to remove himself entirely from the drug environment. But the weight watcher can neither absolutely avoid food nor completely remove himself from an environment where food is present. He must eat to live. Being exposed to just a little food often triggers the sort of response that would send an alcoholic or an addict on a month-long binge. (See "The 'Carboholic Strainer' Theory," pages 37 and 38.)

Herein lies the dilemma of the American dieter: "How do I stop when I've had enough—even of good nutritious food?"

Knowledge alone does not usually produce behavior change. However, once we have determined to change our behavior, we need information to help us make rational choices. We need knowledge in order to formulate the values that will guide our lives.

A Little Nutrition With Your Weight Control, Please!

Even the most enthusiastic calorie-conscious dieter may overlook some basic nutritional concepts. A reduction in caloric intake generally reduces the total amount of food an individual consumes. Unless he carefully considers the nutrient content of the foods he does eat, the dieter may easily cheat his body of essential vitamins and minerals. The desire to look slim and attractive can often backfire if these nutrients are as severely restricted as calories.

Please, add a little nutrition to your weight control!

Nutritional deficiencies combined with calorie restriction can cause fatigue and a general run-down feeling. This feeling, in turn, depletes your zest and enthusiasm for your weight-control program, and before you know it, you're off again on the dangerous cycle of yo-yo dieting. If you are informed about the interrelation of nutrition, calories, activity, and behavior, you will be able to sustain a quiet, steady motivation that will endure through the traumas of losing weight.

Some of the more revolutionary plans generate fireball enthusiasm, as they motivate you to burn up large fat reserves. What actually happens on quick weight-loss plans is that there is a significant loss of protein and of large quantities of water—not a healthy approach for sustained dieting. But usually the motivation to pursue them burns out quickly. Perhaps this is nature's method of self-preservation, since prolonged adherence to these poorly balanced diets would be hazardous to your health.

NUTRIENT SHORTCOMINGS IN THE AMERICAN DIET

While it is difficult to generalize about nutritional deficiencies in the American diet, recent studies indicate certain trends. A ten-State survey conducted among a representative cross section of population by the Department of Health, Education, and Welfare indicated that a significant percentage of the people studied manifested some nutritional difficulties. Iron deficiency was found throughout, but was most severe in low-income black males and females.

Most American dietary surveys show that the following nutrients are frequently deficient in the diets of most age groups: calcium, vitamin A, iron (in women), and vitamin C.

Calcium is by far the most abundant mineral element in the body. About 99 percent is concentrated in the bones and teeth. Calcium combines with other minerals to help give the skeletal system its strength.

Dairy products account for approximately three fourths of the calcium in the average American diet. If on your diet you are avoiding milk, cheese, yogurt, and ice cream, you will require a high intake of foods such as collards, turnip greens, mustard greens, kale, and broccoli in order to fulfill the recommended adult requirement of eight hundred milligrams of calcium per day. Even on a restricted calorie intake, milk products should not be omitted from the diet, since they provide significant amounts of calcium, as well as many other essential and worthwhile nutrients.

Vitamin A is needed in only very small amounts. Large quantities of this vitamin can be stored in the liver and in fat tissues, so a daily intake is not really necessary. Vitamin A helps your eyes maintain normal vision in dim light. It also contributes to the quality of skin tissue, and appears to be important in the skeletal growth and the tooth structure during the early developmental years.

A deficiency in this nutrient may manifest itself in poor skin and hair quality. Or you may experience extreme difficulty seeing in the dark, particularly right after a bright light shines in your eyes. Night blindness, medically called nyctalopia, may contribute to a significant number of nighttime automobile accidents.

Vitamin A is found in two forms. Pure vitamin A in concentrated amounts comes from foods such as fish, liver, and oils. Milk, butter, fortified margarine, cheese, and egg yolks also contain large amounts of vitamin A. Carotenes are the other form of vitamin A, and they are available in green or deep-yellow vegetables. Abundant quantities of carotene are found in spinach, turnip tops, beet greens, asparagus, broccoli, carrots, sweet potatoes, winter squash, pumpkin, apricots, peaches, and cantaloupe. Generally, the darker the color of the plant, the more carotene contained therein. When we discard the green outer leaves of lettuce and eat the pale leaves, we throw away significant amounts of vitamin A. Someone has quipped that eating pale lettuce leaves is nutritionally equivalent to eating wet paper towels.

Lack of *iron* is another shortcoming in the American diet, particularly among teen-age girls and pregnant or lactating women. Although the total amount of iron in the body is only about five grams, its function is extremely important. Iron is a basic constituent of hemoglobin, which combines with oxygen and is carried to the tissues for cell metabolism. Even though the body conserves much of its iron stores, a woman may suffer from iron-deficiency anemia if, in her childbearing years, she does not eat foods rich in this nutrient. Scanty menstruation or amenorrhea (missed periods) can be due to inadequate intake of iron.

Dairy products are a poor source of iron. Mothers, particularly nursing mothers, must take care to introduce their infants to iron-rich foods after the first six months of life.

Egg yolks, baked beans, and soybeans are good sources of iron, as are certain fruits, such as peaches, apricots, prunes, grapes, and raisins. Enriched and whole-grain breads and cereals also provide a significant amount of iron.

Interestingly enough, in the past a regular supply of dietary iron came from water running through iron pipes and from cooking in iron pots. Modern "improved" aluminum materials have eliminated this source, so it is now necessary to more carefully select iron-rich foods.

The following list should provide you with many choices of iron-rich sources. If you are deficient in iron, your blood lacks sufficient oxygen to burn up calories for needed energy. This may account for the tired, rundown feeling you experience. A prudent selection of iron-rich foods—raisins, prunes, apricots, nuts, peanut butter, figs, grapes, dates—will help alleviate that feeling.

If you are concerned about the effects on your teeth of the natural sugar contained in dried fruits, it would be advisable to brush your teeth after eating or snacking.

Foods High in Iron[1]

Food	Serving	Mg. Iron
Apricots, dried	5 halves	1.5
Chocolate, bitter	1 square	1.3
Dandelion greens	½ cup	2.3
Dates	3-4	.6
Egg	1	1.4
Figs, dried	2	.9
Hazelnuts	10-12	.6
Kale	¾ cup	1.7
Lentils, cooked	½ cup	2.2
Oatmeal, cooked	½ cup	.7
Parsley	10 sprigs	.4
Peaches, dried	3 halves	1.9
Popcorn, popped	1 cup	.4
Prunes, dried	4	1.2
Raisins	5 Tbs.	1.7
Soybeans, dried	2 Tbs.	2.0
Spinach, cooked	½ cup	1.5
Turnip greens	½ cup	1.8
Walnuts	8-15 halves	.3
Wheat, shredded	1 biscuit	1.1

Vitamin C—ascorbic acid—is another nutrient frequently neglected in the American diet. Vitamin C helps protect the body against infection. This fresh-food vitamin is found in its highest concentration in the pulp and juice of oranges, grapefruit, lemons, limes, fresh strawberries, cantaloupe, and pineapple. Tomatoes and certain nonacidic fresh fruits such as peaches, pears, apples, bananas, blueberries, and watermelon are also sources of vitamin C. Broccoli, Brussels sprouts, spinach, kale, green peppers, cabbage, and even potatoes (white or sweet) considerably enhance one's vitamin C intake.

Perhaps the most logical way to ensure getting a proper daily amount of vitamin C is to have an orange or orange juice, grapefruit or grapefruit juice, for breakfast. Since many Americans skip breakfast, this may in part explain why ascorbic acid is one of the nutrients that tends to be lacking in our diets.

Following are some common nutritional flaws and suggested corrections.

LOW LEVEL OF VITAMINS A AND C, MINERALS IRON AND CALCIUM, AND DIETARY FIBER

All of these nutrients, which are in short supply in the typical Western diet, are found in moderate amounts in the fruit and vegetable group. The consumption of fruits and vegetables, particularly fresh ones, has decreased steadily over the past several decades. By increasing the intake of fresh fruits and vegetables and whole-grain breads and cereals, many of our nutritional flaws would be corrected.

TOO MANY CALORIES FOR OUR LOW LEVEL OF ACTIVITY

As a society, we sit too much. Our collective body weight would benefit from the calorie-burning effect of physical activity, particularly walking. If we were to eat slower and walk faster, our bodies would be in better shape!

You may not need to cut back the amount of food that you eat in order to lose weight and fat. Calories are the key. If you control calories, you can control your weight.

The "secret" is to use more foods that are higher in bulk (water and fiber), and fewer foods that are high in fats and sugars.

TOO MUCH FAT IN THE DIET

The average American eats 42 percent of his calories in the form of fat! That's about 900 to 1,500 calories per day. Over the course of a year the fat we eat adds up to between 100 and 150 pounds! From a nutritional point of view there are very few vitamins and minerals found in fat. Try to use only half of the fat you are currently using. A more reasonable (and healthier) goal would be to keep the total fat intake to 20 to 25 percent of the total calories.

TOO MUCH SUGAR IN THE DIET

The average American eats 105 pounds of sugar per year! That's about 2 pounds of table sugar per week, 32½ teaspoons a day. (This figure does not include corn or maple syrups, honey, dextrose, or molasses. It's estimated that the total sweetener intake is about 128 pounds for every man, woman, and child in the United States!) About 17 percent of our daily calories comes from the sugars, which supply almost no nutrients except calories.

Each level teaspoon of sugar contains 16 calories. (If you use a rounded teaspoon, it's double.) That's 520 calories per day! The majority of those teaspoons of sugar do not come from the sugar bowl, but are hidden in a wide variety of foods. In 1973 the per capita consumption of soft drinks was 27 gallons per year, up more than 100 percent from 1960.

If weight is to be controlled, sugar consumption should be cut in half and kept well under 10 percent of the total calorie intake. Watch out for those hidden sources!

Consumption of sugar can trigger a continued compulsion for the ingestion of more and more sugary products. If there are little or no protein foods being eaten with the sweet foods, a person may experience a "sugar high" followed by a "sugar low" after the insulin processes the initial sugar. Children who have eaten a breakfast of sugar-coated rainbow cereal, imitation orange juice, and jellied white toast often experience that sugar-low, drowsy feeling by ten o'clock.

HIDDEN SUGARS IN FOODS (IN TEASPOONS)

Banana split	25
Malted milk (1 pint)	15
Fruit pie (⅙ pie)	10
Chocolate cake (4-oz. piece)	10
Sherbet (½ cup)	9
Glazed doughnut (1)	6
Macaroon cookie (1 large)	6
Soft drink (8-oz. serving)	5
Rice pudding (½ cup)	5
Jelly, jam (1 tablespoon)	4-6
Chocolate candy (1-oz. piece)	4
Brownie (1-oz. piece)	4
Ice cream (3½-oz. serving)	4
Plain pastry (4-oz. piece)	3
Canned fruit (½ cup)	3
Honey (1 tablespoon)	3
Gumdrop (1)	2
Apple butter (1 tablespoon)	1

TOO MUCH PROTEIN AND TOO LITTLE COMPLEX CARBOHYDRATES

Many well-intentioned dieters have been deceived into believing that those popular quick-weight-loss schemes are beneficial. They may help you lose weight—at least temporarily—and they may keep you from getting hungry, because of the high protein and fat levels. The problem is that these diets don't necessarily burn up fat and that the weight you lose may be only water. If your diet contains too little water and too few carbohydrates, then you will probably experience fatigue, irritability, and dehydration. Be careful.

BREAK-THE-FAST SKIPPERS

Almost all overfat people do one or more of the following:
1. Skip breakfast.
2. Eat too small of a quantity/quality breakfast.
3. Eat a breakfast high in fats/sugars.
4. Eat a breakfast too low in protein.

We are a nation of breakfast skippers. Many of us share the feeling of Towson State University student Sandra Weiner, who admitted, "I know that three meals a day is the healthy way, but I can't eat breakfast on an empty stomach!" Of those who eat something for breakfast, it's often either not enough or too high in fats and/or sugars. If you are really interested in being a success at weight and fat control and in improving your overall diet, health, and life—then seriously consider the following information.

An adequate (and substantial) breakfast provides for 20 percent to 25 percent of your daily nutrient needs. That means almost one fourth of your proteins, minerals, vitamins, *and* calories. A continental breakfast of juice, donuts, and coffee won't fulfill the criteria. Even if you add a bowl of cereal and a slice of toast, it still falls short.

GUIDELINES AND CRITERIA FOR AN ADEQUATE BREAKFAST

1. Plan what you are going to eat before you go to bed.
2. Plan for nutrient density—that is, quality nutrients in few calories.
3. Remember that an adequate breakfast contains 20 to 25 percent of each of the recommended 56 nutrients.
4. Plan for at least one serving from *each* of the four food groups, totaling a minimum of 4 servings. (pages 112 to 117.)
5. An adequate breakfast contains a minimum of 400 calories low in fats and sugars.

6. An adequate breakfast contains a minimum of 12 grams of protein.

PROTEIN CONTENT OF COMMON BREAKFAST FOODS (in grams)

Milk (8 oz.)	9
Cheese (1 oz.)	7
Egg (large)	6
Bagel (egg)	6
Cottage cheese (1 oz.)	4
Peanut butter (1 oz.)	4
Cooked cereal (½ cup)	3-5
Whole-wheat bread (1 slice)	3
White bread (1 slice)	2
Cold cereal (1 oz.)	2

Cold breakfast cereals may supply you with many of the necessary vitamins and minerals; but eaten by itself, a bowl of cereal is a very low-protein breakfast. If you routinely eat cereal for breakfast, also consume supplementary protein foods such as cottage cheese, eggs, peanut butter, or extra milk. Unfortunately, what some cereals lack in protein they make up for in sugar.

Percent of Sugar Content of Commercially Available Breakfast Cereals[2]

Commercial Cereal Product	Sugar Content
Shredded Wheat (large biscuit)	1.0%
Shredded Wheat (spoon-size biscuit)	1.3%
Cheerios	2.2%
Puffed Rice	2.4%
Uncle Sam Cereal	2.4%
Wheat Chex	2.6%
Grape Nut Flakes	3.3%
Puffed Wheat	3.5%
Alpen	3.8%
Post Toasties	4.1%
Product 19	4.1%
Corn Total	4.4%
Special K	4.4%
Wheaties	4.7%
Corn Flakes (Kroger)	5.1%
Grape Nuts	6.6%
Corn Flakes (Food Club)	7.0%
Crispy Rice	7.3%
Corn Chex	7.5%
Corn Flakes (Kellogg)	7.8%
Total	8.1%
Rice Chex	8.5%
Raisin Bran (Skinner)	9.6%
Concentrate	9.9%
Rice Crispies (Kellogg)	10.0%
Raisin Bran (Kellogg)	10.6%
Heartland (with raisins)	13.5%
Buck Wheat	13.6%
Life	14.5%

Thin From Within

Granola (with dates) 14.5%	Super Sugar Crisp. 40.7%
Granola (with raisins) . . . 14.5%	Cocoa Puffs 43.0%
Sugar Frosted Corn Flakes 15.6%	Cap'n Crunch 43.3%
40% Bran Flakes (Post) . 15.8%	Crunch Berries 43.4%
Team. 15.9%	Kaboom 43.8%
Brown Sugar-Cinnamon Frosted Mini Wheats . . 16.0%	Frankenberry. 44.0%
40% Bran Flakes (Kellogg) 16.2%	Frosted Flakes 44.0%
	Count Chocula 44.2%
Granola 16.6%	Orange Quangaroos 44.7%
100% Bran 18.4%	Quisp 44.9%
All Bran 20.0%	Boo Berry 45.7%
Granola (with almonds and filberts). 21.4%	Baron Von Redberry 45.8%
Fortified Oat Flakes 22.2%	Vanilly Crunch 45.8%
Heartland. 23.1%	Cocoa Krispies. 45.9%
Super Sugar Chex 24.5%	Trix 46.6%
Sugar Frosted Flakes . . . 29.0%	Froot Loops 47.4%
Bran Buds 30.2%	Honeycomb. 48.8%
Sugar Sparkled Corn Flakes 32.2%	Pink Panther 49.2%
	Cinnamon Crunch 50.3%
Frosted Mini Wheats 33.6%	Lucky Charms 50.4%
Sugar Pops 37.8%	Cocoa Pebbles. 53.5%
Alpha Bits 40.3%	Apple Jacks 55.0%
Sir Grapefellow. 40.7%	Fruity Pebbles. 55.1%
	King Vitamin 58.5%
	Sugar Smacks 61.3%
	Super Orange Crisp 68.0%

Many people have seemingly reasonable excuses for skipping or eating an inadequate breakfast. "I'm not hungry." "There's not time in the morning." "I don't like typical breakfast foods."

What if you were told that you would never have long-term success on a weight/fat-control program *unless* you ate a nutritionally adequate breakfast? Could you then learn to be hungry? Would you make time? Would you prepare tasty breakfasts? Although I usually refrain from making absolute-sounding statements, I could come very close to one about breakfasts. After working with and interviewing hundreds of overfat people of all ages and backgrounds, I can't remember that one of them was eating an adequate breakfast, according to the criteria already given, before beginning the *Thin From Within* program.

A Little Nutrition With Your Weight Control, Please!

UNDERLYING CAUSES OF SKIPPING BREAKFAST

A late-night snack may tide you over until the next morning, but it may also interfere with your natural desire to eat breakfast. If you are indulging in an after-dinner snack, cut it out. If you're still not hungry in the morning, then cut back on part of your dinner. Yes, breakfast is a more important meal than dinner!

Late-night television viewing can also interfere with breakfast the next morning. If you stay up late, then you may want to sleep in until the last-possible moment. If something is cut out of a schedule, it's usually breakfast. Is the late-night show, the news, or the weather really more important than breakfast? There will be weather tomorrow—whether you like it or not. Besides, when a person watches television he or she is more likely to snack, perhaps out of boredom.

Morning habits could also interfere with eating an adequate breakfast. Smokers claim that breakfast interferes with their smoking. Coffee addicts say that food detracts from the taste of the coffee. Some children (and parents) become so engrossed in morning television that they "forget" to eat. Even healthful and positive habits such as running and praying early in the morning could interfere with eating a nutritious breakfast.

No matter what your excuse, if you're convinced that breakfast is important to you, then you'll *make* the time for an enjoyable, nutrient-dense meal. It will start you out with a solid foundation for having a beautiful day!

If you experience a midmorning drag somewhere between the hours of nine and noon, this sag in efficiency and pep may have a nutritional origin. You usually finish your last meal fairly early in the evening. If you eat breakfast around seven the next morning, you are breaking a fast of at least twelve hours, assuming, of course, that you had no midnight snack before going to bed.

The liver can store only about a twelve-hour supply of sugar (glycogen), and the blood carries a two-to-three hour reserve of glucose. Breakfast is a convenient time to restore and supplement the liver's fast-depleting supply of this source of stored energy. By skipping breakfast, you extend the normal twelve-hour fast, thereby causing a net blood sugar deficiency for several hours. When the blood sugar and liver sugar supplies are both depleted, you are likely to feel fatigue. This usually occurs in late morning.

Furthermore, if there are great physical demands, an individual with an empty stomach will more quickly deplete the liver's supply of glycogen. Physical exertion without an adequate breakfast may cause you to feel dizzy, weak, or even to pass out. If you have noticed this drag, you are probably putting an unnecessary strain on your system by asking your body to extend its normal nightly fast. The brain and nervous system function best when there is an adequate supply of glucose. If your "get up and go" feels like it got up and went, your central nervous system may be trying to tell you something.

If you have been skipping breakfast, it may take several weeks to adjust to the changed routine, but the rewards in increased efficiency will be well worth the effort.

FAST BUT NUTRITIOUS BREAKFASTS

If you plan ahead, breakfast can be prepared in less than five minutes. A hard-boiled egg and a toasted English muffin topped with cheese, served with a glass of orange juice, are an example. Several eggs may be boiled and stored in the refrigerator for quick use. By using the cottage cheese as a topping, there is little need to butter or jelly the muffin. For the economically minded, you might consider reconstituting your frozen juice with an extra half or full can of water. The juice will be of a better consistency, will last longer (or allow you to consume more fluid by drinking more), and will be absorbed faster, because the fructose is less concentrated.

Here is an adaptation of a recipe developed by the

A Little Nutrition With Your Weight Control, Please!

State of Kansas. The unique aspect of this Perfect Breakfast Muffin is that the batter can be stored for up to six weeks in the refrigerator.

PERFECT BREAKFAST MUFFINS
(about 4 quarts of batter)

2 cups boiling water
2 cups seedless raisins
5 teaspoons baking soda
¾ cup shortening
1½ cups brown sugar
6 eggs, slightly beaten
1 quart buttermilk
3 cups whole-wheat flour
2½ cups enriched white flour
3½ cups all bran cereal
2 cups 40% Bran Flakes
1½ cups nuts, chopped
1 teaspoon salt
½ cup wheat germ

Place raisins in a bowl. Pour boiling water over them. Add soda and cool. Cream shortening with sugar. Blend in eggs and buttermilk. Fold in cooled raisin mixture. Sift flour into large bowl. Add cereals, nuts, salt, and wheat germ. Add the liquid mixture all at once to the flour-cereal mixture. Stir and blend until just moistened. Cover and store in refrigerator. It will keep for six weeks. This makes about 4 quarts. When needed, put in muffin tins and bake 20-25 minutes at 375 degrees.

PRAGMATIC NUTRITION

In response to the need for a simple way to deal with human nutrition, the Institute of Home Economics, United States Department of Agriculture, developed categories known as the Four Food Groups. These can be easily adapted to the vegetarian way of life.

This grouping allows for considerable flexibility in food selection. Variety and moderation should be your guiding principles as you select foods from each group. Variety of texture and color in foods, varied methods of preparation contribute to a well-balanced diet and minimize the "food blahs."

The Four Food Groups form your nutritional foundation. Selecting foods as recommended in these groupings utilizes approximately half of the calories required by an adult, while providing all of the protein, vitamin A, vitamin B_2 (riboflavin), vitamin C (ascorbic acid), and calcium necessary to maintain health. Nearly all of the B_1 (thiamin) and niacin will also be supplied.

The greatest deficiency of this guide is that it provides only about one half to three fourths of the iron needed daily by women in their childbearing years. We can build on this Four Food Group foundation by supplementing our diets with foods rich in iron or in whatever nutrients we need.

BREAD-CEREAL (GRAINS) GROUP

Four or more servings daily.

One serving:
> Bread (whole grain, enriched, or nutritionally restored): 1 slice
> Ready-to-eat cereal: 1 ounce.
> Cooked cereal, corn meal, grits, macaroni, noodles, rice, spaghetti: ½ to ¾ cup.

VEGETABLE-FRUIT GROUP

Four or more servings (including requirements for vitamins C and A).

One serving: ½ cup or 4 ounces of fruits and vegetables.

One daily serving of vitamin C from—

Citrus fruit	Cabbage
Strawberries	Potato
Cantaloupe	Salad greens
Tomato	

Every-other-day serving of vitamin A from—
> Dark-green or deep-yellow vegetables: peppers,

broccoli, asparagus, squash, pumpkin, et cetera.

MILK-CHEESE GROUP

Two or more servings daily for the adult.

Children and pregnant women, 3 or more servings; teen-agers and nursing women, 4 or more servings.

One serving:

Milk: 1 cup (8 ounces)

This may be whole, evaporated, or skim milk; reconstituted dry milk, buttermilk, or soy milk.

Cheese: 1 to 1½ ounces American/cheddarlike cheese.

Yogurt: 1 cup (8 ounces)

Cottage cheese: 1½ cups (12 ounces)

Ice cream: 1 pint (16 ounces)

MEAT-ALTERNATIVE GROUP

Two or more servings daily.

One serving:

Eggs: 2 (this includes those used in cooking).

Beans, peas, lentils, garbanzos, soybeans: 1 cup cooked dry beans.

Peanut butter: 4 tablespoons.

Soy cheese, vegetable proteins, and nuts are also included in this group.

Two groups of foods not included in the Four Food Groups are junk foods consisting mostly of "empty calories," such as potato chips, pretzels, candy, soft drinks, sugar, and miscellaneous foods such as coffee substitutes, herb teas, spices, flavorings, herbs, and artificial sweeteners. The miscellaneous group adds a great deal to the overall palatability of the diet without adding significantly to the calories, but neither of these groupings provides appreciable nutrients in relation to your total daily needs. A good rule of thumb to use when selecting foods is Do the calories exceed the nutritive value?

Although the Four Food Groups guide has been

criticized for not meeting all of our nutritional needs, it has the distinct advantage of reducing a very complex biochemical science to a simple practical system that can be understood and remembered. Without restricting your food selection, this approach classifies foods into a practical system that supplies almost all of the fifty-six nutrients needed to maintain your health.

BREAD-CEREAL GROUP

Selections of whole-grain and enriched breads or cereals, as well as rice (brown preferred) and enriched macaroni, noodles, and spaghetti, form the foundation of the daily diet recommended in the Four Food Groups. Whole-grain or unbleached flours, or those enriched with thiamin, riboflavin, niacin, and iron, contribute to the fulfillment of the suggested requirements for these nutrients. Whole-grain breads and cereals utilize the entire kernel, including the nutrient-packed germ as well as the bran. Bran (along with dried fruits, nuts, seeds) is an excellent source of dietary fiber, an essential component for good health.

The *Thin From Within* program strongly recommends using whole-grain breads and cereals. These have more vitamins, minerals, protein, and fiber than the white or dark-colored breads. Whole-grain products also stay with you longer, thereby delaying hunger. Don't be enticed into thinking that dark breads are whole grain. Many manufacturers are adding caramel coloring to white flour to give the illusion of a whole-grain bread. Read the label to set a better table.

The following chart identifies the nutrients that are removed during the milling process in order to make white bread or dark-colored white bread.

PERCENTAGE LOSS OF NUTRIENTS IN PROCESSING OR REFINING OF WHEAT

Biotin (B vitamin)	90
Vitamin B_1 (Thiamine)	86
Niacin	86

Iron	84
Phosphorus	78
Copper	75
Magnesium	72
Manganese	71
Folic Acid (B vitamin)	70
Vitamin B_2 (Riboflavin)	70
Vitamin B_6	60
Pantothenic Acid (B vitamin)	54
Calcium	50

Only vitamin B_1, vitamin B_2, niacin, and iron are added in the enrichment process.

Perhaps one of the most palatable and psychologically rewarding of foods is homemade bread. The sight, smell, and texture make the eight-to-twelve-minute kneading process an enjoyable activity. Yeast breads are particularly intriguing. Mixing flour, yeast, salt, and water can result in the most flavorful Italian bread. Simple breads such as this are surprisingly low in calories. Even a strong-willed person has trouble resisting seconds or thirds of fresh homemade bread.

VEGETABLE-FRUIT GROUP

There are two special requirements regarding the four daily servings recommended from the vegetable and fruit group:
1. One serving should come from a citrus fruit or other source of vitamin C daily.
2. To help fulfill the vitamin A requirement, at least every other day one serving should come from a dark-green or deep-yellow-colored vegetable.

Two other servings of any vegetables and fruits, including potatoes, will round out this group.

Just because a person is on a calorie-restricted diet, he need not eliminate potatoes. This vegetable, particularly when prepared whole and consumed with the skin, provides important nutrients. The more surface area exposed in preparation—that is, the smaller the pieces are cut up or sliced—the fewer the nutrients. The potato's most significant supply of nutrients lies just under the skin. Sweet potatoes supply significant quantities of vitamin A, plus additional iron. Generally, it is what we put on the potatoes—butter, margarine, sour cream— that makes the calories mount. Eaten plain and whole, the potato can be a worthwhile, tasty diet component.

On a health-promoting weight/fat-control program, you are reminded that a diet containing many fruits and vegetables will allow you to eat a larger amount of food and still consume fewer calories. Because of their bulk, foods from this group will also fill you up.

MILK GROUP

Many important nutrients such as calcium, riboflavin, protein, and other minerals and vitamins are found in appreciable amounts in milk in its various forms.

However, it is important to point out that there is more to good nutrition than just drinking milk. There is no perfect food, not even a nearly perfect food. Sometimes a milk lover will fill himself up with milk, crowding out many other good foods. Often children drink their milk before eating and then claim they are too full to eat the meal. However, by the time dessert is served, they claim they're hungry! They are not lying. The fact is that this perfect timing occurs because the all-liquid diet moves out of the stomach in five to fifteen minutes—which correlates nicely with dessert time.

The following chart suggests the quantity of other calcium-containing foods that would have to be consumed to equal one serving, or eight ounces, of milk.

CALCIUM EQUIVALENTS OF EIGHT OUNCES OF MILK

1½ oz. cheese
12 oz. ice cream
12 oz. cottage cheese
3⅝ lbs. carrots
3⅜ lbs. cabbage
12 eggs

5 large grapefruit
6 oranges
10 lbs. potatoes
½ to ¾ lb. of kale, turnip, or mustard greens
2 lbs. broccoli or cooked green beans
¾ lb. endive
4 lbs. green peas

In choosing milk and milk products and their alternatives, you may want to consider, in addition to the calcium content, the price and the calories.

Skim milk	90 calories
1 percent butterfat milk	115 calories
2 percent butterfat milk	140 calories
Whole milk, 3.5 percent butterfat	160 calories

MEAT-ALTERNATIVE GROUP

The foods in the meat-alternative group provide the bulk of high quality protein. Protein molecules are made up of smaller building blocks called amino acids. There are 22 amino acids, 8 of which are essential for adults, and 9, possibly 10, of which are needed by infants and children during growing spurts. An essential amino acid is one that the body cannot synthesize or manufacture from its basic chemicals. A *complete* protein provides the individual with all 8 of the essential amino acids. These must be supplied directly from the diet if normal growth and development are to take place.

Lean cooked beef, veal, lamb, poultry, and fish are all concentrated sources of complete protein. But meat sources are the most expensive sources, and also the highest in calories per serving. Muscle fibers of meat are laced with fat particles, the most concentrated source of calories. If you eat large servings of meat daily, excessive protein calories can make you just as fat as excessive carbohydrate or starch calories.

For the vegetarian, the many available varieties of beans, dried peas, lentils, and nuts, including peanut butter, can function in combination to fulfill the necessary protein requirements. Two eggs constitute a serving of high quality protein.

Americans generally consume excessive quantities of meat. Currently a movement to minimize meat consumption is having an impact on our country. Proponents of this movement suggest that many of earth's labors are squandered. To provide prime meats we feed our cows grain that could be feeding our human populations. Cattle may consume as much as twenty pounds of grain for each pound of edible return.

The "meat" group is more than just what meets the eye. There are many nutritious nonmeat alternatives that will supply the necessary nutrients common in the meat group. Vegetarianism is a viable low-calorie/low-fat alternative for the nutrition-minded weight watcher. Chapter 9 covers the basics of vegetarianism.

FOUR FOOD GROUPS SUMMARY

For the adult the jingle to remember is "4-4-2-2 is sound nutrition for you." (For children use 4-4-3-2; teen-agers, 4-4-4-2.) These are minimums. You can eat more than the minimums without getting too many calories.

Group I (Grains): 4 servings per day.

Group II (Vegetables-Fruits): 4 servings per day.

Group III (Milk-Cheese): 2 servings per day.

Group IV (Meat Alternatives): 2 servings per day.

PERSONAL DIET STUDY

One of the best ways to determine the nutritional adequacy of your diet is to do a long-range diet study. This involves a considerable amount of paper work, since you must record *all* the foods that go into your mouth. The following forms have been provided for this purpose. It would be beneficial to do this personal diet study periodically to keep a check on the nutritional adequacy of your diet. It's a lot of work but well worth it for the insight you will get into your actual nutritional patterns.

On the form at the top list all the foods you have

A Little Nutrition With Your Weight Control, Please!

Daily Food Intake

Foods Consumed	Approx. Amount Consumed	Calories
Breakfast		
Lunch		
Dinner		
Snacks		

Checklist

_____
verdict

FOUR FOOD GROUPS ANALYSIS		
	One check per serving	Total Calories for Each Food Group
Bread-Cereal (Grains) Group (4)		
Vegetable-Fruit Group (4) One check for each fruit or vegetable **C** for each vitamin C source **A** for each vitamin A source		
Milk-Cheese Group (2)		
Meat Alternates Group (2)		
Empty Calories		
Miscellaneous		

consumed during the day (breakfast, lunch, dinner, and snacks); how much of each you have eaten; and how many calories each food amounted to. In order to do this you will need to purchase a good calorie-counting book. Pocket-sized editions are fine. Use this to supplement the information in the charts on pages 74 to 81. Be sure to include *everything* you have taken in, however insignificant—mustard, catsup, onions, sugar, butter, jelly, chewing gum, et cetera. The goal is to be as complete and as accurate as possible. So often a dieter fails to accurately guesstimate the size of each serving. A diet scale takes the guess work out of dieting.

The form at the bottom is a simplified Four Food Groups checklist. For each food item that you consume, you should check some column on this side of the form. Even junk foods such as candy, and miscellaneous foods such as catsup, should be noted and checked. If you eat more or less than one suggested serving, record the appropriate fraction consumed. For example, 4 ounces of milk = ½ a serving.

For the vegetable and fruit group, give yourself a check for *every* one of these foods you eat. Then, if the food is a source of vitamin C (such as citrus fruits, tomatoes, strawberries), also place a **C** within the subdivision of the vegetable and fruit group. Similarly, dark-green and deep-yellow-colored vegetables (such as string or wax beans, spinach, corn, kale, peas), which are rich in vitamin A, should be noted by an **A** within the subdivision. But remember, *all* fruits and vegetables—including those marked as rich sources of vitamin A and vitamin C—should be checked in the top part of the vegetable and fruit box.

If you have fulfilled your Four Food Group requirements for the day (4-4-2-2) draw a smile on the face on the top-right-hand side of the form. If not, draw a frown. If you're not sure, reread the chapter.

Do not change your normal eating patterns while you are carrying on the study. For this period only, try not to modify your diet to comply with the Four Food Groups. If

A Little Nutrition With Your Weight Control, Please!

you do, you may defeat the purpose of studying your nutritional pattern. Your goal is to find out what you normally eat.

Keep a checklist for the next three days. Run a similar check at least four times a year.

Circle all the fats and sugars in your diet with a red-colored marker. Write a summary statement about the quality of your diet in your diary. Were you able to gain any insight into your eating patterns? What modifications in your life style are in order?

---

[1] Adapted from Mayo Clinic *Diet Manual,* 3d edition (Philadelphia: W. B. Saunders Company, 1961), pp. 188, 189.

[2] From the *Journal of Dentistry for Children,* September-October, 1974.

THE BASICS OF VEGETARIANISM

The average American consumes about 250 pounds of meat per year. Between 35 to 40 percent of the adult population of meat eaters have a weight problem. In contrast to the meat-and-potatoes person, the vegetarian usually has less of a problem with excess weight. Perhaps that's because the vegetarian consumes fewer calories in fat forms from animal sources.

It's estimated that 35 percent of the fat in a traditional diet comes from the meat that people eat. Since fat is the most concentrated source of energy and very low in nutrients, it would behoove our weight-control program to reduce the intake of unnecessary fats. Meat is high in unnecessary fats. On the other hand, it is also high in nutrients. For many years people thought that because meat was high in nutrients it was indispensable in the diet. *No single source of food,* including meat, *is indispensable for human growth and health.* The body requires individual nutrients, not individual foods. Nutrients are best found in a wide variety of foods.

The United States as a nation has come to rely heavily on meat, perhaps too heavily. When asked, "What's for dinner?" the questioner waits until the meat course is mentioned. Because meat has a high-nutrient density, people erroneously believe that they have covered all of their nutritional needs by eating it. That's not true. Meat can be a *part* of adequate nutrition, but it's far from a perfect food. Because of its fat content, the meat group contains more calories per serving than does any other food group. In consuming meat you get the bad with the good, the unneeded fat with the needed nutrients. Because meat is not nutritionally indispensable and because you are better off without those unnecessary fat calories, you might want to consider a change to a lower-fat vegetarian life style. If you decide to eliminate unnecessary fat calories by eliminating meat, how do you get the nutrients that meat once provided?

WHAT IS A VEGETARIAN?

Some people believe that vegetarians eat only vegetables. They say, "Oh, I could never be a vegetarian; I don't like vegetables!" George Bernard Shaw in his witty way with words retorts: "A vegetarian is no more one who eats vegetables than a Catholic is one who eats cats."

The word *vegetarian* sounds as if it comes from the word *vegetable,* but, in fact, it was derived from the Latin word *vegetus,* which means "sound, whole, fresh, lively." Perhaps this provides a better explanation of why most vegetarians prefer to use whole-grain products, fresh fruits, and vegetables.

As a working definition, the word *meat* is used in this chapter to refer to the flesh, muscle, and or organs of any animal that walks, crawls, swims, or flies.

ALTERNATIVES AVAILABLE TO THE VEGETARIAN

Years ago a person was considered to be either a meat eater or a vegetarian. Today the choice isn't that simple. In fact, you might even be able to label many people as two thirds of a vegetarian. It just seems to be a matter of degree. For example, if someone eats meat only once a day then he is two thirds of a vegetarian. However, most omnivorous Americans would not view

themselves as an "almost vegetarian," nor would practicing vegetarians readily welcome two thirds of a vegetarian into their membership. No doubt many meat-eating people have gone for days without meat. An omelet
for breakfast, peanut butter sandwich for lunch, and a
cheeze pizza for dinner might not even be recognized as
a meatless day by the average American.

On the other side, a pure vegetarian is very difficult to
find. If the term is defined as one who does not consume
animals or animal products, then this too becomes a
matter of degree. Most all food supplies, even the air and
water, contain microscopic organisms that are part of the
animal kingdom. Some of our grains, seeds, nuts, and
spices come to us with insect parts and rodent hairs—
compliments of the FDA![1] Yet some vegetarians are so
against the consumption of animal products that they will
strain the gnats out of their lemonade. With the above as
a backdrop, vegetarian alternatives range from the more
restrictive to the more liberal in food selection:

Fruitarian consumes only the fruit portion of the plant
(including seeds and nuts). This alternative is often
selected for short periods during a juice fast.

Vegan eats whole-grain products, fruits, vegetables,
nuts, seeds, beans, and peas, but consumes no milk
products or eggs. The vegan has high reverence for
all animal life and therefore does not use products
made or derived from animals.

Pure vegetarian selects the same types of food as the
vegan, abstaining from milk products and eggs, although fortified soy milk may be used.

Lactovegetarian allows for the use of milk products—
including milk, cheese, yogurt, and ice cream—as
well as the grains, seeds, fruits, vegetables, beans,
peas, and nuts.

Ovovegetarian uses eggs but no milk products. Food
selection also includes the standard vegan fare.

Lacto-ovovegetarian includes the use of both milk products and eggs, plus plant foods.

Pisces vegetarian (with or without lacto/ovo) eats plant

products and fish (and other animal products from the sea).

Poultry vegetarian (with or without lacto/ovo) uses plant products and chicken, turkey, other domestic fowl, and/or game birds.

Pisces-poultry vegetarian (with or without lacto/ovo) consumes, perhaps it is safe to say, just about everything *except* red meats.

The alternatives from which to choose are many. There are advantages and disadvantages to each alternative. A word of caution should be given for health and safety. Unless you have a sound grasp of the field of nutrition that will enable you to get a well balanced diet, the more restrictive alternatives are not recommended.[2]

This chapter is unabashedly biased toward the lacto-ovovegetarian alternative. In spite of the unresolved controversy currently raging in regard to cholesterol in eggs, the lacto-ovovegetarian alternative seems to provide the greatest flexibility in preparation, the widest variety of nonmeat foods, and the best balance of nutrients.

Some vegetarians use meat analogs, or textured vegetable proteins (TVP)—products that have been developed to look, and in even some cases to taste, like beef, chicken, or pork. Some people when they make the transition from a meat to a vegetarian life style have found these soybean-based TVP products helpful. When other ingredients are added to the soybean base (wheat, corn, milk, or egg white), the textured vegetable protein foods can have the same protein efficiency ratings as real meats.[3]

REASONS FOR CHOOSING A VEGETARIAN DIET

Among the many reasons for choosing a vegetarian life style, the following present only a sample, and are by no means meant to be a complete listing. One or more of these reasons may influence a person to choose to follow a vegetarian diet.

Religious/Spiritual. Some religions encourage vegetarianism. A few have adopted vegetarian alternatives as the official church position. Some individuals have chosen vegetarianism for various spiritual reasons. Others feel led by the Scriptures or other spiritual writings to choose a vegetarian life style.

Humane/Ethical. This viewpoint maintains that life is sacred. There is a special reverence for life in general—and in specific, all animal life. To sacrifice the life of a living creature for food is unethical—particularly when many viable alternatives exist in most societies.

Health/Fitness/Medical. This point of view suggests that most people would be far healthier if they chose not to eat meat. They might even live longer. Vegetarians have less heart disease and cancer. Recent research has demonstrated that carcinogenic properties (cancer-producing substances) are carried in animal fat.[4] When one makes the transition from a meat to a nonmeat life style, he increases his usage of whole-grain products, fresh fruits, and vegetables. This, in turn, increases the fiber and bulk of the diet, which increases the frequency of bowel movements.

There also tends to be a quid pro quo (this for that) effect operating in the life of a vegetarian. As the person tunes into health through diet, he also becomes more concerned about his related health behaviors—smoking, alcohol consumption, sugar consumption, and physical-fitness level.

Ecological. When we eat meat we are eating high on the food chain. Animals, particularly cattle, are fed grains that could be used for food by humans. Much of the edible lower-priced foods are squandered on the bovine and could be better put to use by feeding people. Cattle can manufacture sufficient protein from eating grass; they don't need to eat grain.[5]

Economic. Meat products cost more per pound than many high-protein alternatives. If a person is economically oriented, he learns quickly that cutting the consumption of meat results in lower grocery bills.

Your reasons for choosing to follow a vegetarian life

style may involve a combination of several of the above categories. All of these may somehow have influenced you in this direction. Whatever your reasons, you need to grow in your understanding and appreciation of them if they are to become a strong motivating factor in changing your life style.

NUTRITION FOR THE VEGETARIAN

Nutrients are the building blocks of sound nutrition for both the meat eater and the vegetarian. There are about fifty-six of these that are needed by the human. The body doesn't require any particular food. It just needs the nutrients. The cells don't care what foods or combinations of foods bring them the nutrients so long as the nutritive substances are available in their proper amounts when the cells need them. Recommended daily requirements have been suggested by the National Academy of Sciences for most of the fifty-six nutrients.

The nutritional needs of the meat eater and of the vegetarian are identical. The differences are in the foods and food combinations that are chosen by the vegetarian and the nonvegetarian to get the materials that the cells require.

The list of recommended nutrients in a healthy diet is awesome. It would take a brain like a nonlinear computer to remember all the substances, the recommended amounts, and then what foods had how much of which nutrients. Fortunately the entire process has been simplified by the Four Food Grouping arrangement (see pp. 112-118). Remember, we're interested in supplying our body cells with the optimal level of nutrients through the foods that we choose to eat. The *nutrients* are the end goal, not the foods. The food groupings have been devised with nutrients in mind. If certain foods in a grouping do not appeal to you, then choose from the alternatives suggested.

The easiest way to cover your nutritional needs would be to select at least one serving from each of the Four Food Groups at each meal. Your protein needs (both quantity and quality) would be covered with a minimum of hassle.

PROTEIN COMPLEMENTARITY

Man cannot live by bread alone, nor can he live by vegetables alone. Variety and moderation appear to be the most sensible guidelines for a healthy life style. These two guidelines are also apropos for protein nutrition for the lacto-ovovegetarian. The greater variety of foods from which the vegetarian selects his meals, the more likely it is that the meal will be nutritionally adequate.[5]

Protein Basics. The human body needs to manufacture quality proteins to support life. Because the flesh of animals contains quality proteins, for years people have illogically deduced that they must eat the quality proteins in animal flesh if their bodies are to make the quality proteins to support human life.

Proteins are made up of amino-acid building blocks. All proteins contain from 8 to 18 different amino-acid combinations. There are literally hundreds of thousands of different proteins in both the plant and animal kingdoms, containing millions of amino-acid combinations.

There are eight amino acids that the human body cannot synthesize (make from the chemical elements). These eight are called *essential* or *indispensable,* because the body cannot make them and thus must get them through the food supply. Meat and animal products (milk and eggs) contain all eight of these amino acids in their proper balance to support human growth. Most plant products also contain all eight, but not in the proper balance to support growth when eaten by themselves. Most plant products have one or more essential amino acids in limited amounts, which limit the plant proteins' effectiveness to support human growth, if eaten alone. These "limiting amino acids" are usually lysine in grains, methionine and tryptophan in legumes, and some combination of the three in nuts and seeds.

Nutritionally, the body doesn't care whether you supply it with high quality protein from an animal source or from several complementary plant protein foods eaten together at the same meal. What the body ultimately needs is all of the amino-acid blocks readily available in their proper amounts. These can be easily supplied by eating two or more combinations of grains, milk products, seeds and nuts, or legumes at the same meal.

In the book *Diet for a Small Planet*, Frances Moore Lappe presents an excellent detailed discussion of protein complementarity. She gives specific examples and recipes for the many complements between grains and milk products; grains and legumes; legumes and seeds. Lappe also shares a limited number of protein complements between legumes and milk products; grains and seeds; and milk products and seeds.[5]

Adequate nutrition for the vegetarian is not difficult to obtain. It is similar to that of the meat eater but with special emphasis on protein and iron.

Iron. The best sources of dietary iron are the red meats, followed by some of the nonred meats. These sources contain heme iron (from the blood of the flesh), which appears to be more readily absorbed in the intestines than nonheme iron (23 percent of the heme iron is absorbed as contrasted with 3 to 8 percent of the nonheme iron). About 60 percent of the iron found in meats is of the nonheme variety. Unlike heme iron, its absorption is less efficient and influenced by the other foods with which it is ingested.[6]

Grains, fruits, vegetables, nuts, legumes, seeds, and the nonflesh animal products (eggs, cheese, milk) contain only this less-efficiently absorbed nonheme iron. Nonheme iron absorption can be enhanced by the presence of ascorbic acid and/or the presence of animal tissue (flesh, but not eggs, milk, or cheese).

Therefore, the vegetarian seems to be at a minor disadvantage in iron absorption. Furthermore, most vegetarians consume a diet high in fiber, which may also bind up some of the iron and make it unavailable for absorption. Vegetarians are recommended to keep a

careful nutritional eye on their iron intake, planning regularly for iron-rich meals with ample vitamin C, to enhance the availability and absorption percentages.
The following chart lists iron sources for the vegetarian.

IRON SOURCES

Mg. Iron	Food	Amounts
10.5	Prune juice	1 cup
7.9	Black beans	1 cup cooked
7.7	Mung beans	1 cup cooked
6.9	Garbanzo beans	1 cup cooked
6.1	Pinto beans	1 cup cooked
6.0	Baked beans	1 cup
5.1	Lima beans, dry	1 cup cooked
5.1	Navy beans	1 cup cooked
4.9	Soybeans	1 cup cooked
4.8	Rice bran	¼ cup
4.4	Rice polishings	¼ cup
4.3	Lima beans, green	1 cup cooked
4.2	Lentils	1 cup cooked
4.0	Spinach	1 cup cooked
3.9	Millet	¼ cup dry
3.9	Peaches, dried	5 halves
3.6	Turnip greens	1 cup
3.4	Split peas, green	1 cup cooked
3.2	Molasses, blackstrap	1 Tbs.
2.9	Peas, fresh	1 cup
2.8	Beet greens	1 cup cooked
2.8	Blackeye peas	½ cup frozen
2.8	Chocolate, sweet	3½ oz.
2.6	Chard	1 cup cooked
2.6	Raisins	½ cup
2.4	Dates	10 medium
2.3	Dandelion greens	½ cup cooked
2.3	Tofu	4 oz.
2.2	Shredded wheat	2 biscuits
2.2	Tomato juice	1 cup
2.0	Pumpkin seeds	2 Tbs.

1.9	Snap beans, green	1 cup cooked
1.9	Wheat bran	¼ cup
1.9	Wheat germ	¼ cup
1.8	Figs, dried	4
1.8	Kale	1 cup cooked
1.8	Mustard greens	½ cup cooked
1.8	Prunes	5 cooked
1.8	Soybean milk	1 cup
1.7	Brussels sprouts	8 cooked
1.6	Broccoli stalks	2 large, cooked
1.5	Apricots, dried	5 halves
1.5	Strawberries	1 cup
1.4	Egg	1 large
1.4	Oatmeal	1 cup cooked
1.4	Potato	1 large, cooked
1.2	Mushrooms	6 large

One of the problems with consuming foods rich in iron is that, for the most part, they are high in calories. Persons following restricted-calorie meal plans often fall short of the recommended daily allowances for iron (males, 12 mg; females in their childbearing years, 18 mg). The average American diet, including meats, contains about 6 mg of iron per 1,000 calories. Therefore the average American woman on an average intake of 2,000 calories would still be 6 mg, or 33 percent, short of her recommended iron allowance! Restricted-calorie diets compound the problem. If she goes on a 1,200-calorie diet, she may consume only about 7.2 mg of iron—only 40 percent of her recommended daily allowance! With great care in food selection from iron-rich sources, the woman on a restricted calorie diet can have an adequate iron intake.

Eggs and Cholesterol. In the 1950's cholesterol was singled out as a causative factor in heart disease. In the 1960's triglycerides were implicated, then linked with cholesterol as contributing factors. In the 1970's HDL's (high-density lipoproteins) were in the coronary limelight.[7] Perhaps in the 1980's some of the *real* culprits will be exposed—stress, sedentary life styles, obesity, high blood pressure, smoking, and the consumption of alcohol and caffeine in excess.[8]

For the high-stressed, physically inactive American, cholesterol *may* be *one* causative factor in coronary heart disease. But is it the excess cholesterol or other factors that are more important? The human body manufactures between 70 and 80 percent of the cholesterol found in the bloodstream. Stress causes the body to produce more—far more—than normal dietary ingestion. If your dietary intake of cholesterol is low, the body will produce more.[9]

Physical inactivity allows excess cholesterol to accumulate in the body. Regular, vigorous physical activity helps keep the cholesterol levels in check. (Such activity also helps reduce stress by allowing an outlet for pent-up emotions. Physical activity may also help reduce both blood pressure and obesity.) Diets with higher-than-average fiber contents will help move excess cholesterol out through the stools.

A cholesterol-restricted diet may change readings by 20 percent (even though there could be up to a 15 percent plus or minus error in the readings), but lowered cholesterol levels have not been helpful in reducing the incidence of heart disease. Prior to the blood sampling, fasting is recommended for 8 to 12 hours, but there is evidence that a 14-hour fast is more accurate.[8]

Until further evidence is available, perhaps it would be prudent to look at all the risk factors for heart disease in your life before you make a decision about how many eggs are "healthy." If you are under stress, physically inactive, overweight, and smoke—then maybe you shouldn't eat eggs. The fewer risk factors you own, the more eggs you can safely eat. If you're a normal weight, non-smoking, jogging-fitness fan, with a high-fiber vegetarian diet, low-stress life style—then you could probably safely eat a moderate number of eggs per week—and still have safe cholesterol readings.

Graphically this could be represented by plotting your fitness level against your leanness level. The higher your fitness-leanness level, the more cholesterol you can safely ingest. The lower that level, the less dietary cholesterol would be recommended.

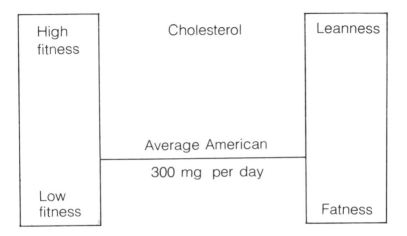

The average American is generally unfit and overfat. It is recommended that he limit his cholesterol intake to between 250 and 300 mg per day.

SUMMARY OF VEGETARIANISM

Adequate nutrition is not difficult for the lacto-ovovegetarian.

Adequate protein quality can be obtained by—

Eating at least one serving from all Four Food Groups at each meal.

Consuming a milk/cheese/yogurt serving with other foods at each meal.

Complementing the amino-acid balance of grains/legumes/seeds/milk products at each meal.

In order for protein complementarity to be effective the proper balance of amino acids must be consumed at each meal.

Thin From Within

Vitamin B$_{12}$ is not a problem for the lacto-ovovegetarian.

Select whole-grain breads and cereals.

Use fresh fruits and vegetables when available.

Do not overcook your vegetables. Use a minimum of water, to preserve the nutrients. .

Choose foods that are rich in iron.

Eat from a wide variety of foods and food groupings, but be moderate in the amounts you select.

Continue to read and learn about some of the more intricate details of vegetarianism.

Experiment in the kitchen with tasty food combinations.

[1] "The High-Filth Diet, Compliments of the FDA," *Consumer Reports,* March, 1973.

[2] "Nutrition and Vegetarianism," *Dairy Council Digest,* vol. 50, no. 1 (January-February, 1979).

[3] R. G. Stoia and N. Martin, *Adventures in Dining: A Vegetarian Gourmet Cookbook* (Kettering, Ohio: Kettering Medical Center, 1978).

[4] *Life and Health, Vegetarianism* (Washington, D.C.: Review and Herald Publishing Association, 1973).

[5] Frances Moore Lappe, *Diet for a Small Planet,* revised edition (New York: Ballantine Books, Inc., 1975).

[6] Elaine E. Monsen, "Simplified Method for Calculating Available Dietary Iron," *Food and Nutrition News,* vol. 51, no. 4 (March-April, 1980).

[7] "'Good' v. 'Bad' Cholesterol," *Time,* Nov. 21, 1977.

[8] Edward R. Pinckney and Cathey Pinckney, *The Cholesterol Controversy* (Los Angeles: Sherbourne Press, 1973).

[9] "Cholesterol Metabolism," *Daily Council Digest,* vol. 50, no. 6 (November-December, 1979).

THE ROLE OF ACTIVITY IN WEIGHT CONTROL

There is no doubt that inactivity is an important factor in the frequency of "creeping overweight" in our modern Western societies.

According to English law, life does not begin until "quickening" occurs. Quickening is the first recognizable movement of the fetus in the uterus, and it generally happens around the fourth or fifth month of pregnancy. From quickening until death, movement is a sign of life; it is basic to our existence.

Man alive is man in motion, but the less we move, the less we desire to move. Eventually we develop patterns of inactivity that, once established, are extremely difficult to change. The majority of people today are hypokinetic—we don't move enough. We ride rather than walk, sit rather than stand, and lie down rather than sit. This love of ease can lead to "dis-ease."

BATTLING THE LAW OF INERTIA

Our highly mechanized and automated society places such a high value on saving steps that movement has come to seem almost unnatural. Have you ever gone for a walk and been offered a ride by friends driving past? When you graciously declined their offer, did they become insulted or look at you as if you were crazy, because you'd rather walk?

If you hope to become and remain active, you may have to plan ahead for the activities that you enjoy. As activity becomes a regular part of your normal daily routine, it becomes less awkward. But the first step is the hardest. Our habitual desire to remain inactive may make it necessary to do something radical to break the pattern.

A basic law of physics suggests that a body at rest tends to stay at rest. The human body at rest has an additional restraint—the brain. Thanks to our higher level of consciousness, we can think up ingenious rationalizations and excuses for why one's own particular body should stay at rest. We must constantly wage war against this indolent intelligence if we ever hope to enjoy the many benefits of the active life.

Here are a number of motivational quotes that may help you overcome the inertia of your body at rest:

If you're not using your body, you're not using your head.

Exercise builds your life, not just your body.

You can't push a button for good health, but you *can* push yourself away from the table.

Give yourself a gift: add better years to your life by adding more life to your years.

THE DOUBLE BIND OF INACTIVITY

Most dieters try to lose weight only by cutting their caloric intake. Unfortunately, the body may interpret a diminution of calories as a famine, and react by slowing down the metabolism. Conversely, when activity level increases, the body reacts by increasing the metabolic rate, figuring that food must be just around the corner. This increased metabolic rate is maintained for about twenty-four hours. Therefore, the active person is burning up more calories even while asleep than is his friend who has restricted his food intake but is sedentary.

The Role of Activity in Weight Control

Paradoxically, inactivity can *increase* the appetite. There appears to be a regulatory center in the hypothalamus area, called the appestat, that balances caloric intake and expenditure. This appestat becomes functional only when an individual remains moderately active. The appestat is not sensitive enough to deal with extremes. If too little activity is engaged in, the balance it normally maintains is thrown out of kilter. For the hypothalamus area to function properly, the body needs to be in motion a total of 40 to 60 minutes each day.

The overweight individual requires more calories than an individual of normal weight to do the same task. It's as if he were carrying a weight strapped around his waist. The system is overloaded by excess poundage, and he requires more energy to do the same amount of work. This may be the major reason for the cyclic nature of inactivity and overweight.

As a person becomes less active, which usually happens after he finishes school, the appestat is thrown out of kilter. He eats slightly more and begins to gain weight, because of inactivity and excessive eating. This combination puts weight on faster than either factor would working alone. As the individual's weight increases, it takes greater effort to engage in even simple movements. As the difficulty of exerting effort increases, activity levels decrease, and the appestat remains jammed. Now the person is overeating more than ever.

Eventually the individual tends to become stabilized at the overweight, inactive level. Stabilization occurs when calories used balance out the number of calories consumed. Because he is carrying an extra load, the overweight person needs to consume an enormous number of calories to give him enough energy to maintain his restricted activity.

This ball-and-chain effect keeps the individual inactive, because his overweight condition makes even minimal effort fatiguing. You can verify this by deliberately overloading your own system the next time you take a walk. Fill your pockets with rocks or carry a small child.

After several minutes of walking you will begin to get the point. But don't stop there. Be sure to walk up a flight of stairs to get the full effect of carrying excessive weight. You will see what the overweight individual experiences with every movement he makes. The only exception is in the swimming pool. Fat makes one buoyant, so the more overfat a person is, the fewer calories he expends to keep himself afloat!

EXERCISE VERSUS ACTIVITY VERSUS MOVEMENT

The word *exercise* often connotes a physical education class in which a group of people do jumping jacks, sit-ups, and push-ups to the cadence set by the drill instructor. That is one form of movement, but few of us would choose calisthenics as the activity we most enjoy. I prefer the term *activity,* which conjures up fewer negative associations. Activity, in turn, is based on movement. The more we move, the more active we are. And to be physically fit, we must be very active indeed.

Many people who claim they are active actually move very little. "How do you get your activity?" "Oh, I play tennis." Yet, if you observe the average person on the court, you will probably notice that he swings only if the ball is hit right to him. He rarely moves his feet, and consequently is hardly active at all. Calories consumed in playing a set of tennis vary tremendously, depending upon how much and how vigorously the person moves. The hit-it-right-to-me player might better be designated as playing *at* tennis.

ACTIVITIES

Make a list of your favorite activities.

Indicate next to each activity how much you engage in it daily or weekly.

Star the ones that involve a considerable amount of movement—the way *you* participate.

Place a double star next to those activities that involve a great deal of movement utilizing the large leg muscles.

The Role of Activity in Weight Control

Movement is more than just a periodic workout. Movement should become a pattern of life. We need to assess the degree to which we move and figure out ways to move more if we hope to increase our caloric expenditure.

Unfortunately some have confused fitness with activity for keeping in check one's fatness. There are many physically fit persons who are still fat. They work out thirty minutes each day and sit or lie down the other twenty three and one-half hours. For controlling one's fatness, total movement time is the key. Walking is one of the best fat-controlling activities. Add some "leg power" to your life style.

ACTIVITY, ADOLESCENTS, AND ADIPOSE TISSUE

"Instead of merely counting the calories a fat girl consumes, obesity experts are now translating her daily activity into calories—that is, finding how much energy she uses up in a day, and how this balances with the energy she takes in as food (which is also measured in calories). By observing fat girls swimming, playing volleyball, taking gym, they have learned that these girls remain remarkably motionless. In the swimming pool they are likely to do a dead man's float while others are practicing their crawl. Lack of activity explains why a girl who doesn't eat excessively can still become fat. If two teen-agers of the same weight eat equal amounts of food, the one who takes a half-hour's brisk walk daily will be in the neighborhood of fifteen pounds lighter at the end of a year.

"During the teen years boys typically slim down while girls gain more fat. The probable explanation is that boys are increasing their physical activity while girls are decreasing theirs almost to the vanishing point. Gym periods, often held only twice a week, give a girl a bare ten minutes of actual exercise, and many, pleading menstrual discomfort, manage to skip gym frequently. The experts believe that differences in exercise habits explain why city girls are plumper than those from rural areas and why Massachusetts girls weigh more than those from sunny California."[1]

1. Do you feel that your excess poundage is due to excessive calorie intake, lack of appropriate, regular activity, or a combination of both?
2. When you engage in various activities, are you an active or passive participant? How do you know?
3. Do you generally get out of breath after brief, fairly strenuous activity?
4. Do you mind sweating?
5. List several common-sense ways of increasing your activity patterns.

MISUNDERSTANDINGS ABOUT ACTIVITY

1. *To affect your weight, the activity must be concentrated.* It *is* true that to lose one pound of body fat—3,500 calories—a person would need to chop wood for 7 hours, play volleyball for 11 hours, walk 35 miles, or climb the Washington Monument 15 times! Based on this, people rationalize that if it requires so much effort to lose one pound of body fat, then it is not very realistic to include activity in their weight-control plan. If one uses the same logic, however, calorie restriction would not make sense either, since an enormous amount of food would have to be eliminated in order to lose one pound of body fat. We know, of course, that this is not true—the effects of calorie restriction are *cumulative*. Well, so are the effects of activity.

   It is not necessary to do all the activities in one continuous bout, any more than it would be to try to lose a pound a day through dieting. A man could chop wood for 30 minutes a day, and in 14 days he would lose one pound of body *fat* (not water from sweat). A person could walk one mile per day, and in approximately one month lose one pound of body fat, provided his eating habits and other activities remained unchanged. This realistic but moderate change in physical activity would result in a 12-pound weight-loss per year!

2. *An increase in activity also means an increase in appetite.* Since many people eat out of sheer boredom, it would almost be more true to say that a decrease in activity means an increase in appetite. Actually, it is the balance between what is taken in and what is expended that is most crucial to weight control. After several hours of vigorous activity the appetite of the sedentary individual might actually decrease.

Too inactive a life appears to throw the normal balance of eating and activity out of kilter. Research has demonstrated that when a sedentary individual engages in at least a half hour of vigorous physical activity, his appestat becomes more accurate in regulating his food intake.

BREAKING THE CYCLE OF ACTIVITY RESTRICTION

Most of us are locked into a cycle of activity restriction. Our philosophy of doing things the easy way is so deeply ingrained into our lives that we may not even be aware of its pervasive influence.

If you make a conscious effort, this cycle of activity restriction can be interrupted. Friends, books, personal determination, values reassessment—any or all of these may motivate you to begin an activity program. After about six weeks of increased activity you'll actually begin to experience a rejuvenation of physical and psychic energy! You will have developed endurance and increased your tolerance to the buildup of lactic acid, an end product of metabolism that can cause the feeling of fatigue. Further motivation to maintain the increased activity levels will come from your friends, who will make encouraging comments about the changes they observe.

WALKING: AN ANTIDOTE TO TENSION

"Tension is probably the most widespread complaint that people bring to their physicians. It gives them headaches, backaches, elevated blood pressure. It keeps them awake at night or tossing in unrestful sleep. It makes them inefficient at work and irritable at home. They take expensive pills and go on expensive vacations to get rid of their tension. They win relief for a while, but the tension is always there, stealing back into muscles and nerves and tying body and mind into little knots.

"Walking is the direct physiological answer to tension. Even a short brisk walk can drain away anger and anxiety, solve a problem, untangle the knots both physical and psychological. Walking as a regular part of the day or week draws off tensions before they turn into headaches and insomnia that need pills, or backaches that take expensive orthopedic skills to relieve them.

"Most people do not know that walking, commonplace ordinary walking, can perform these wonders for them. Or if they have been told, they do not believe it. Yet it is a relatively simple interaction of body and mind, psychosomatic and somatopsychic, which does not require a course in physiology to understand. The mechanisms by which walking restores and preserves muscular, nervous, and emotional health are a heritage as ancient as the first man."[2]

1. What techniques do you currently use to relieve tension?

2. Have they consistently worked?

3. Have you ever tried walking as a tension antidote?

4. Would you consider *regular* walking if you believed it could serve as a preventive factor against tension, irritability, and insomnia?

5. Do you believe a regular program of walking can do the things suggested in No. 4?

6. What plan would you be ready to undertake with regard to walking?

SPOT REDUCTION

Many people wish to reduce specific areas of their bodies without necessarily affecting the remaining areas. Isolated fat reduction is almost impossible to accomplish.

Adipose tissue is deposited throughout the body in a pattern that is common to most people. Although each individual has his own distinctive pattern, the following order of fat deposition generally applies: hips, buttocks, thighs, waist, chest, upper arms, face, and fingers.

To the disappointment of most dieters, weight also comes off in a predetermined manner, which is generally the reverse order from the way it went on: fingers, face, upper arms, chest, waist, and lastly, thighs, buttocks, and hips.

Many women ask, "How can I reduce in all areas of my body except my breasts?" Unfortunately, there is no answer; breast shrinkage may be one of the noticeable results of a weight-loss program.

For the most part, doing trunk exercises will not reduce excessive fat deposits around the trunk but it will firm up the underlying muscles. Walking will not burn up fat only in the thigh area. The fat burned up by physical activity is drawn from stored-up deposits throughout the body; some of it even comes from the deeper tissues rather than from the tissues immediately under the skin.

LOSING INCHES BUT NOT POUNDS

Activity programs that isolate specific groups of muscles may not effect a *weight* loss, but can be of great benefit in reducing fat, particularly for relatively inactive individuals. Even though your scale may show no change, you will profit both physiologically and psychologically from activity.

Muscles respond to increased activity by gaining not only in strength but also in tone and weight. The toned muscle holds larger quantities of blood protein. As the muscle tones up, the flabbiness is lost, and you may lose

143

Thin From Within

inches around the muscle without losing any weight. This is because of the increased denseness of the toned fiber, which contains much more fluid than a flabby muscle. If you are interested only in weight loss, this could be discouraging. However, losing inches and fat is as important to your health and appearance as losing weight. You will feel trimmer. Your clothes will hang differently and your muscles feel tighter. People will begin to comment that you've lost weight—even though you know better. So don't become discouraged because the scale is not cooperating. Believe in how you look and feel! Enjoy the new, active you!

One important group of muscles is the abdominals, which in Americans are notoriously weak. The pot belly needn't, but too often does, characterize middle age. We tend to avoid movements that would strengthen these muscles. Walking and running don't do much for the abdominals. Sitting for long periods of time further weakens this muscle group. Up until recently, sit-ups have been thought to strengthen the abdominal muscles. Recent findings, however, suggest that straight-leg sit-ups are only minimally effective in strengthening them; most of the effort of a sit-up strengthens the hip flexor muscles in the back rather than the abdomen.

However, there is a way of performing sit-ups so as to benefit the abdominal muscles. Instead of lying with your legs stretched out, bend them at the knee, either by keeping your feet close to your buttocks or by placing your calves on a chair or bench. Now, do your sit-ups from this position. People who may perform well with straight-leg sit-ups find that their performance of bent-leg sit-ups is markedly reduced—often by more than half. Another alternative is the bent-leg sit-back. S-l-o-w-l-y sit back from the full bent-leg sit-up position.

The strengthening and toning of the abdominal muscles will not necessarily cause you to lose significant stores of fat around the abdominal area. Fat loss results from a caloric deficit. What you will notice is a reduction in your waist size. Many individuals claim a waist reduction of two or more inches within a month or less just from consistently doing sit-ups with their legs bent.

BENEFITS OF A PROGRAM OF ACTIVITY

The rewards of breaking out of the passivity and inertia that characterize most Americans can be great. As hard as it may be to start and stick to a regular program of activity, once you have determined upon it, it will become easier and easier to continue in it as the physical, psychological, and social gains make themselves apparent. When you feel better in body and mind, when people begin to respond to you more positively, you will find that you are so full of energy and good will that you will actively enjoy your new life style.

PERSONAL BENEFITS FROM ACTIVITY

Keep a written record of every benefit you have derived from a more active life. List the date you began each activity, and the date you first noticed each benefit.

FROM MOVEMENT TO FITNESS

Would you like to be able to go through a normal day's routine without undue fatigue, and still have energy left in reserve with which to meet emergency situations? Then you are interested in physical fitness. Physical fitness comes from movement, but not just any old kind. Movement with a purpose enables you to utilize larger quantities of oxygen in a given period of time, which results in greater biological efficiency.

You may have broken out of your cycle of movement restriction. You may even have developed a movement orientation to life. But most likely you are still not physically fit. The achievement of physical fitness requires a concentrated effort to fully utilize every movement, to derive from it the maximum potential.

---

[1] Alice Lake, "Obesity," *Seventeen Magazine*, October, 1969, p. 129.
[2] Aaron Sussman and Ruth Goode, *The Magic of Walking* (New York: Simon & Schuster, Inc., 1967), p. 27.

THE SPIRITUAL ASPECTS OF WEIGHT CONTROL

The spiritual component of becoming thin from within may present the most important challenge in this book. Our spiritual self is that part of us that makes us uniquely special. For some reason we tend to hide our spiritual beauty from most people and allow it to be known only by a few intimate others. Sometimes we become so overly protective of our spiritual essence that we negate its importance in helping us achieve the fullness of life.

In the area of weight control we need all the help we can get! To approach a weight-control program without considering the power of the spiritual is like trying to drive a car without one spark plug. It's a jerky stop-and-go journey at best, and few who try it ever reach their destination without some kind of problem.

The spiritual is open to many interpretations and may rightly mean many different things. The spiritual can be understood to mean one or more of the following:[1]

1. A unifying force *within* the individual.
2. That which gives meaning or purpose to life.
3. A common bonding force *between* individuals.
4. An individual belief, faith, perception (in or of a "transcendent other").

The Spiritual Aspects of Weight Control

Spiritual power, strength, and energy are thought to be available from three sources:
1. Within oneself.
2. From others.
3. From God.

All three sources of spiritual power have something to offer. The first two have their limits, but power from God is limitless if we consistently choose to seek it. When we use all three available sources of spiritual power, we develop a stable triangular base for spiritual strength.

Oneself. Tapping into the power available within may momentarily give us the ability to handle whatever comes our way. It can help us stick to the tasks at hand with singleness of mind and spirit. However, when the negative elements of life come—disappointment, rejection, discouragement, criticism, guilt, and failure—they can break the spirit. When we're really down and feel sorry for ourselves, we could care less about weight control or attempting to live a thin-from-within life style. If we are to properly use the strength from within, we need to get rid of the negative thinking that can eventually break our spirits.

Others. Other people, singly or in groups, can share spiritual energy with us. When in the presence of certain people, we can almost feel that specialness, that esprit de corps, that they exude. Tapping into their power, we become renewed and revitalized. New alternatives and vistas of experience open before us. Our own sense of self-worth and specialness is enhanced. But significant "others" also have their limitations. People move and change. At certain points in our lives, we outgrow our need for groups that once were important to us. At such times we need to look, even search, for new support groups and significant people who can help us grow.

God. When we tap into God's power, we draw from an eternal, never-failing wellspring—a source of spiritual power we can always depend on. As we do so we begin to sense the awesomeness of His creative power. We sense the fact that there is order in the universe. We realize that God is in control. We become more confident in and responsive to His care and unconditional love. We begin to appreciate the parent nature of God and His willingness to extend His power and energy to His children—that power which can cause even the improbable to become possible for us.

Weight control has much in common with spiritual faith. We can read books about it, talk about it, go to meetings, join groups, but until we *live* it—daily—it probably won't make a lasting difference in our lives. To be committed implies more than an occasional passing thought. In a sense, to be committed to weight control or spiritual faith is similar to a love commitment. Scores of thoughts remind us of our commitment. We look for meaning in the mundane that can apply to what we prize. We relate much of what we daily experience to our commitment. In other words, success in relationships, spiritual development, and even in weight control doesn't just happen. Success is the result of increased knowledge, daily practice of the basic principles we have accepted, and assertive confrontation of problems that arise (sometimes with the help of a counselor). Such success requires ongoing work. When we let up, so does progress.

Often in life we tend to go at it alone. Perhaps our egos suggest that we can accomplish our goal by our own effort. The facts are that in weight management 57 percent of the adult population are out of control. Going at it alone for many Americans means going fat. In weight management we need all the help we can get.

Books, lectures and workshops, weight-control clubs and self-help groups, friends and family, doctors and counselors, all are part of the sources we need in order to be successful at weight control. But when we've tried them, when we've "been there," and the fat is still with us—then what do we do? Where do we turn? Perhaps that's when we need a Power that transcends oneself and others—not as a last resort, but as a genuine acknowledgment of our often unrealized need for God and

His power to guide our lives. But if spiritual faith hasn't yet made much of a difference in our personal fat control, then it may not have made much of a difference in any other part of our lives either.

When our spiritual development has given us enough evidence, then we'll be ready to let go and let God guide our eating activity, and behavior. As long as we try to control faith and fat, we will undoubtedly fall short of our goal. But as we let go and let God guide, we can achieve any goal. God created us, knit us together in our mothers' womb. He knows our needs—completely (Psalm 139).

Temples of God. When we attune ourselves to God and His will, we begin to appreciate that what He created and what we have given anew to Him (our bodies) is special and sacred. Our bodies become the temple of God's Spirit (1 Cor. 6:19). Like everything else we think we own, we are really "on loan" from God. We're asked to be manager's of another's property—stewards of our bodies. Are we good managers of God's property? Does God's Spirit live in a well-nourished, sturdy temple, or is the body temple sagging with excess fat from too many calories and too little activity?

PRACTICAL SPIRITUAL SUGGESTIONS FOR SUCCESSFUL WEIGHT CONTROL

- Begin each day with spiritual attunement. Ask God to grant you some of His power to help you apply sensible weight-control guidelines to your life.
- Realize that prayer won't melt the fat off your hips, but it can change your attitudes so that God's power can be applied to your personal weight-control program.
- Keep a spiritual diary on your insights regarding your personal growth as it relates to weight control.
- Before you eat *each* meal or snack, ask God to bless the food; ask Him for the strength to limit your caloric intake to the preplanned portion; ask God for the wisdom to help you slow down your eating speed.
- After (or during) the meal, take a minute to thank God

for providing you with the food, wisdom, strength, and alternatives.

● While planning, selecting, and preparing meals, ask God for guidance; then focus attention on preparing low-fat, low-sugar, high-nutrient-density meals.

● Periodically during the day allow yourself the privilege of a few moments of meditation—focusing on God's goals for your life.

● Invest some regular time in creative imagery. See yourself by God's grace actually controlling what has been the major obstacle to reaching your weight goal.

● Focus some time each day on one attribute of God. Believe that, since you're a child of God, you are entitled to a portion of that attribute. Here are a few suggestions: beauty, compassion, creativity, energy, goodness, wonder, harmony, joy, light, love, order, patience, truth, serenity, peace, grace, glory, trust, silence, will, wisdom, forgiveness, stillness, balance, awareness, friendship, security, hope.

SUMMARY STATEMENT

Your spiritual belief can be an integral part of your weight-control program. It's really not necessary to try first all the weight-control techniques before you turn to God's program for your life. Sometimes we can get so wrapped up in worrying about every detail of life that we lose sight of our life priorities. But Scripture reminds us: " 'So my counsel is: Don't worry about *things*—food, drink, and clothes. For you already have life and a body—and they are far more important than what to eat and wear. . . . Will all your worries add a single moment to your life?' " [2]

" 'Set your heart first on his kingdom and his goodness, and all these things will come to you as a matter of course. Don't worry at all then about tomorrow. Tomorrow can worry about itself! One day's trouble is enough for one day.' " [3]

We who are spiritual have the blessed hope of eternal life, but let's not overlook the beautiful life that we can now lead with God. The great Christian symbol of the cross easily encompasses all our burdens and struggles. From the emptiness of the tomb, we too are called to a resurrection—a victory—over our struggles. We, too, are called to celebrate the fullness of life. As Jesus said: "'I have come that men may have life, and may have it in all its fullness.'"[4] May God bless you in your journey through life.

---

[1] Rebecca Banks, "Health and the Spiritual Dimension: Relationships and Implications for Professional Preparation Programs," *Journal of School Health,* vol. 50, no. 4 (April, 1980), pp. 195-202.

[2] Matt. 6:25-27; from *The Living Bible,* copyright 1971 by Tyndale House Publishers, Wheaton, Ill. Used by permission.

[3] Verses 33, 34, from J. B. Phillips: *The New Testament in Modern English,* Revised Edition. © J. B. Phillips, 1958, 1960, 1972. Used by permission of Macmillan Publishing Co., Inc.

[4] John 10:10; from *The New English Bible.* © The Delegates of the Oxford University Press and the Syndics of the Cambridge University Press 1961, 1970. Reprinted by permission.

SUMMARY GUIDELINES FOR BECOMING THIN FROM WITHIN

These guidelines are to be read at least once every day for the next ten weeks. Each day, select one guideline to focus and concentrate on.

ENJOY EATING

Eating is an enjoyable process. Take time to notice the taste, texture, and temperature of the food. Concentrate on the pleasures of eating wholesome foods.

EAT SLOWLY

Take small bites and thoroughly chew each morsel. In order to increase the joy of eating, you must eat slowly. Taste buds are in the mouth, not the stomach.

CONCENTRATE ON EATING

Give food your undivided attention. Do not eat while watching television, reading, or standing. Do not talk with food in your mouth. Do not wash down food with a liquid.

PROPER NUTRITION IS IMPORTANT

Nutritional adequacy is closely related to successful weight control. Proper food selection on a reduced-calorie program will not only help maintain health but also provide a feeling of fullness and increased vitality.

EATER'S MOTTO

"Eat first what your body needs [nutrient density]. Then, if calories allow, what your mind desires."

PLAN DAILY

Plan not only for calorie-controlled, nutritionally adequate meals but also for enjoyable physical activities that will help maintain vim, vigor, and vitality. In other words, plan to really *live.*

THREE MEALS A DAY

Three calorie-controlled meals a day help keep the fat away. Hunger is better controlled with breakfast, lunch, and dinner.

SLIP UPS

It is OK to slip occasionally; it is not OK to feel guilty. Slipping may not be serious so long as you know how to make the appropriate adjustments in your program without sacrificing nutritional adequacy. As time goes on (and you continue to use your mistakes as a learning experience) you will slip less frequently and become more comfortable in the program.

CORRECTIVE MEASURES

Anything consumed over and above the daily caloric allotment must be earned through additional physical activity. A vigorous walk of about 20 minutes burns up 100 calories.

DAILY PHYSICAL ACTIVITY

Activities such as vigorous walking use up a significant number of calories when practiced regularly. At least 20 minutes a day is reasonable. Physical activity can also help regulate the appetite, tone up sagging muscles, and contribute to improved health.

CALORIES DO COUNT

All overly fat people have consumed more calories than their bodies could use. Excess calories are stored in fat tissue. To lose fat, you must use these stored calories, gradually. To assure a healthy and steady fat loss, consume 750 calories less than your body needs each day, and lose one and one-half pounds of fat per week.

COUNT YOUR CALORIES

Calories are, at best, approximations. Don't be a calorie-fraction-counting fanatic. Round off food calories to the nearest 5. Learn to estimate portion size by calorie content.

CONCENTRATED AND REFINED FOODS

Limit your intake of high-calorie foods. These foods are generally high in calories and low in nutrients. Most of these junk foods are concentrated calories in the form of unnecessary fats and sugars.

PRINCIPLES OF WEIGHT CONTROL

Short of surgery there are three choices: 1. Consume fewer calories. 2. Become very active physically. 3. Do a little of both. Choice No. 3 is by far the most beneficial for permanent weight control and continued health.

THE HUMAN BODY IS EXQUISITELY LOGICAL

It's impossible to cheat or deceive the human body. Dishonesty in the mind will show up on the hips. Do not become discouraged if a significant weekly weight loss does not show up on the scales. The body adjusts its water balance according to its own timetable; therefore, weight may not come off steadily. Maintain your faith in the program and persist throughout this water adjustment period.

WEIGHT CONTROL IS LIFELONG

Common-sense, health-conserving weight control means a lifelong program of sensible nutrition and activity. The rule to follow is "If I can't live with it (for the rest of my life), I won't start it."

CHOOSE FROM ALTERNATIVES

Be on guard for situations that make you feel trapped, ashamed, or guilty. Search out reasonable alternatives. Believe in the motto "There *must* be a better way!"

ASSERTIVENESS

Consistently state and practice what you think and feel. Practice living an assertive life style rather than letting someone else control your life.

ACCEPT RESPONSIBILITY

As long as you believe that someone else is responsible for your problems, you will never get rid of them. Do not *use* other people or situations as an excuse. Accepting responsibility for your own behavior is a winning attitude. Repeat the statement "I like the feeling of being a winner."

DO IT! FOLLOW THE PLANS

The greatest plans and programs will not work for you unless *you* do them. An old Chinese quote states:

What I hear, I forget.
What I see, I remember.
What I DO, I know.

SUMMARY

Throughout this book I have been committed to the concept of total (holistic) health. Total health embraces the concept that all six aspects (faces) of the human are important for full, productive functioning. This holistic model (called the SEPISS theory) suggests that all six faces of being fully human, fully alive—Social, Emotional, Physical, Intellectual, Sexual, and Spiritual—intertwine with one another. These components when taken collectively give humans their uniqueness and fullness.

In the area of weight control each component also has its uniqueness. The more of the six faces that are incorporated into your weight-control program, the greater will be your success at staying thin from within. Several of the "learnings" summarized below have interconnections with other faces of the holistic self. You may wish to add your own discoveries to this list.

SOCIALLY, we learned that in weight control—
    Meal-management techniques are important.
    We need to be in control of our sensory cues such as the smell and sight of food.
    It is imperative to plan ahead for nutritiously satisfying meals.

It is important to plan ahead for calorie-controlled snacks.

Physical activity must be planned for in advance, just like our meals.

We need to become comfortable when assertively saying No! to ourself and others.

EMOTIONALLY, we learned that in weight control—

Certain behavior-modification techniques can be helpful in managing our eating environments.

Certain value-clarification strategies can help us get in touch with what we sense as being important to us.

Some of our negative thinking can keep us "thinking fat," which prevents fat from coming off the hips.

Positive thinking and imagery can help in keeping us focused on our goals.

How we choose to invest our time reflects our priorities—the things that we really value.

There are many ways to deal with our emotional ups and downs, but first we might profit from putting our emotion through the NETS. Is the emotion (1) Necessary? (2) Edifying? (3) Truthful? (4) Self-serving?

Our belief system has a tremendous influence on our eating, activity, and behavior.

PHYSICALLY, we learned that in weight control—

There is great value in *daily* physical activity in regulating the appetite and in calorie expenditure.

A nutritionally sound breakfast will provide a nutritional advantage in our weight-control program.

Adequate nutrition can be acquired through fewer calories if we keep the sugar and fat to a minimum.

Regular, consistent nutrition and daily physical activity when carefully planned ahead will keep us from getting hungry.

Thin From Within

INTELLECTUALLY, we learned that in weight control—
The head can win the "battle of the bulge."
Success is a matter of mind over platter.
Calories DO count and to lose weight we need to use
up more calories than we take in.
There are an unlimited number of alternatives that we
could employ for success, but each one
begins with us and our willingness to "DO IT!"
We can be successful—if we want to be.

SEXUALLY, we learned that in weight control—
Physical attraction is still a reality of life—period.
Many people want to lose weight—be more physically attractive—for reasons of fashion or
whatever. (Advertisements play this idea to the
hilt!)
Sexual attraction is real and powerful, and can be
used in a proper way to help us reach our
goals.

SPIRITUALLY, we learned that in weight control—
We need all the help we can get.
We have spiritual resources inside ourselves.
Disappointment, discouragement, and failure can
break our spirit.
A spiritual belief system gives meaning to the
rhythms of life.
All other faces of the holistic self intertwine around
the spiritual.
Hope, strength, energy, and fortitude originate in the
spiritual.
There is a Power greater than ourselves that we can
tap to make the impossible possible.
The spiritual area can be cultivated and can grow.

BIBLIOGRAPHY

Bailey, Covert. *Fit or Fat? A New Way to Health and Fitness Through Nutrition and Aerobic Exercise.* Boston: Houghton Mifflin Company, 1978.

Berland, Theodore. *Rating the Diets.* Skokie, Ill.: Consumer Guide, 1974.

Bruno, Frank J. *Think Yourself Thin: How Psychology Can Help You Lose Weight.* New York: Barnes and Noble Books, 1972.

Cooper, Kenneth. *Aerobics.* New York: Bantam Books, Inc., 1968.

———. *The Aerobics Way: New Data on the World's Most Popular Exercise Program.* New York: M. Evans and Company, Inc., 1977.

Cooper, Mildred, and Kenneth Cooper. *Aerobics for Women.* New York: Bantam Books, Inc., 1972.

Danowski, T. S. *Sustained Weight Control: The Individual Approach.* Second edition. Philadelphia: F. A. Davis Company, 1973.

Ewald, Ellen Buchman. *Recipes for a Small Planet: High Protein Meatless Cooking.* New York: Ballantine Books, Inc., 1973.

Ferguson, James M. *Habits, Not Diets: The Real Way to Weight Control.* Palo Alto, Calif.: Bull Publishing Company, 1976.

———. *Learning to Eat: Behavior Modification for Weight Control.* Palo Alto, Calif.: Bull Publishing Company, 1975.

Katch, Frank I., and William D. McArdle. *Nutrition, Weight Control, and Exercise.* Boston: Houghton Mifflin Company, 1977.

Kuntzleman, Charles T. *Activetics: 297 Ways to Lose Weight Painlessly Without Dieting.* New York: Peter H. Wyden, Publisher, 1975.

Lappe, Frances Moore. *Diet for a Small Planet.* Revised edition. New York: Ballantine Books, Inc., 1975.

Life and Health. Obesity: You CAN Lose Weight. Washington, D.C.: Review and Herald Publishing Association, 1974.

———. *Vegetarianism.* Washington, D.C.: Review and Herald Publishing Association, 1973.

Mahoney, Michael J., and Kathryn Mahoney. *Permanent Weight Control: A Total Solution to the Dieter's Dilemma.* New York: W. W. Norton and Company, Inc., 1976.

Mayer, Jean. *Overweight: Causes, Cost, and Control.* Englewood Cliffs, N.J.: Prentice-Hall, Inc., 1968.

Noland, Jane Thomas. *Laugh It OFF: How Making Light of Your FAT Can Help You Get Serious About Losing Weight and Find Your THIN Self Under All Those Puffy Pounds.* Minneapolis: CompCare Publications, 1979.

Pinckney, Edward R., and Cathey Pinckney. *The Cholesterol Controversy.* Los Angeles: Sherbourne Press, 1973.

Ploeger, JoAnn. *Day by Day: A Dieter's Diary of Homework.* Port Huron, Mich.: Slim Living, 1977.

Robertson, Laurel, Carol Finders, and Bronwen Godfrey. *Laurel's Kitchen: A Handbook for Vegetarian Cookery and Nutrition.* Berkeley, Calif.: Nilgiri Press, 1976.

Rubin, Theodore Isaac. *The Thin Book: By a Formerly Fat Psychiatrist.* New York: Pinnacle Books, 1966.

Shedd, Charlie W. *The Fat Is in Your Head: A Lifestyle to Keep It Off.* Waco, Tex.: Word Books, 1977.

Simon, Shirley. *Learn to Be Thin: The Secret of Permanent Weight Loss Through Behavior Modification.* New York: G. P. Putnam's Sons, 1973.

Stuart, Richard B., and Barbara Davis. *Slim Chance in a Fat World: Behavioral Control of Obesity.* Champaign, Ill.: Research Press Company, 1972.

Stunkard, Albert J. *The Pain of Obesity.* Palo Alto, Calif.: Bull Publishing Company, 1976.

Sussman, Aaron, and Ruth Goode. *The Magic of Walking.* New York: Simon and Schuster Inc., 1967.

Westin, Jeane Eddy. *Break Out of Your Fat Cell: Holistic Mind-Body Guide to Permanent Weight Loss.* Minneapolis: CompCare Publications, 1979.

———. *The Thin Book: 365 Daily Aids for Fat-Free, Guilt-Free, Binge-Free Living.* Minneapolis: CompCare Publications, 1978.

Wyden, Peter. *The Overweight Society.* New York: William Morrow and Company Inc., 1965.

Wyden, Peter, and Barbara Wyden. *How the Doctors Diet.* New York: Pocket Books, Inc., 1972.